Differentiating for Inclusion

Target Ladders:
Working Memory and Auditory Processing

Kate Ruttle

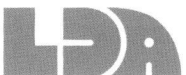

Permission to photocopy

All rights reserved. This book contains materials which may be reproduced by photocopier or other means for use by the purchaser. The permission is granted on the understanding that these copies will be used within the educational establishment of the purchaser. The book and all its contents remain copyright. Copies may be made without reference to the publisher or the licensing scheme for the making of photocopies operated by the Publishers Licensing Society.

The right of Kate Ruttle to be identified as the author of this work has been asserted in accordance with Sections 77 and 78 of the Copyright, Designs and Patents Act 1988.

Target Ladders: Working Memory and Auditory Processing

ISBN: 978-1-85503-612-3

© Kate Ruttle 2017

Illustration on p. 75 © Robin Lawrie

This edition published 2017

10 9

Printed in the UK by Page Bros, Norwich

Designed and typeset by Andy Wilson for Green Desert Ltd

LDA, 2 Gregory Street, Hyde, Cheshire SK14 4HR

www.ldalearning.com

Contents

Introduction: Closing the gap	5
Working memory and auditory processing	8
What is working memory?	10
Implications of poor working memory	11
What is auditory processing?	13
Implications of auditory processing difficulties	15
Working memory difficulties, APD and other specific learning difficulties	17
Diagnosis	19
Creating a working memory- and APD-friendly classroom	24
Supporting children who have working memory difficulties	25
Supporting children who have APD	29
Supporting children who have attention difficulties	30
Supporting children who have poor language development	31
Supporting children who have social difficulties	32
Using Target Ladders	
How to use this book	33
Records of Progress	38
The Target Ladders	
Aspect 1: Auditory processing and exploring sound	42
Aspect 2: Auditory processing for phonological development	48
Aspect 3: Auditory processing for communication	54
Aspect 4: Auditory memory	60
Aspect 5: Visual-spatial memory	66
Aspect 6: Kinaesthetic memory	72
Aspect 7: Memory, attention and organisation	78
References	84
Links to other *Target Ladders* titles	85

All websites were correct at the time of going to press.

Closing the gap

Schools are committed to meeting the needs of children with Special Educational Needs and Disability (SEND). However, the range and complexity of needs encountered in mainstream primary schools continues to grow. The responsibility of identifying the needs, and of supporting class teachers in meeting those needs, lies with Special Educational Needs Co-ordinators (SENCOs), many of whom are class teachers themselves with limited experience of a wide variety of SENDs.

The Children and Families Act 2014 and the Special Educational Needs and Disability Code of Practice 2015 (CoP) both emphasise the importance of high aspirations for children with SEND. One indicator of the 'overall effectiveness' of a school will always be the extent to which the school meets the needs of pupils with SEND. Even if children are not formally recognised as having SEND, the school should still be able to provide evidence of action and intervention for those who are falling behind. School inspectors look for evidence that schools are working to 'close the gap' for all pupils who are not achieving age-related expectations. The first step in closing the gap is to identify what learners can do.

Case study

Gina is in Year 3. Her writing target for two terms has been *'to write well-structured stories'*. The teacher explained that Gina's work was 'all over the place' and he wanted her to write stories with a beginning, middle and end. An exploration of Gina's written work, however, shows that in addition to writing disorganised texts, her basic sentence structure is muddled. Since she doesn't use punctuation, her teacher hadn't noticed this before.

When Gina is asked to retell a story told to the class, it quickly becomes apparent that she hasn't grasped the point of the story and she doesn't understand how events link. Instead, she talks about individual ideas that have caught her attention, flitting from one idea to the next as she recalls something else.

The target *'to write well-structured stories'* is not helpful to Gina because it doesn't accurately identify her difficulties and is not a useful next step. Gina's new targets are *'to sequence three pictures to tell a story'* and *'to reorganise words to make simple sentences'*.

Whether individual targets are recorded on an internal target sheet, a Record of Progress (RoP), a Pupil Passport or some other mechanism, the fact remains that children with SEND continue to need 'small steps' targets in order to clarify learning priorities and give them a sense of achievement when they tick off another target.

The SEND Code of Practice stresses the importance of teachers having a good understanding of individual SENDs and of using their best endeavours to ensure that a child with SEND gets the support they need. The *Target Ladders* series focuses on one SEND at a time, in order that the range of difficulties and challenges facing young people with that SEND can be acknowledged. A child does not, however, need to have a SEND to be helped by the targets and strategies mentioned in the book. If any child in your care has any of the behaviours or difficulties addressed by the book, then the targets and activities should be helpful and appropriate.

The *Target Ladders* series aims to support you by:

- focusing on what a child can do, rather than what they cannot do, in order to identify next steps;
- presenting 'small steps' targets for children;
- suggesting strategies and activities you may find helpful in order to achieve the targets;
- giving you the information you need to use your professional judgement and understanding of the child in determining priorities for learning;
- recognising that every child is different and will follow their own pathway through the targets;
- giving you an overview of the range of difficulties experienced by children with a particular SEND. Not all children will experience all of the difficulties, but once you know and understand the implications of a SEND, it gives you a better understanding as to a child's learning priorities.

Setting useful targets for a child can be tricky, but the process can be simplified if the exploration focuses on what the child *can* achieve rather than what they are not able to do. Once you know what a child can do, you are in a good position to set targets and consider interventions.

Case study

Caleb's Year 5 teacher feels frustrated because Caleb doesn't appear to be making progress in any curriculum areas. Looking back at progress made in previous years, it is apparent that he has been capable of achieving age-related expectations but his progress seems to have halted. One of his peers unwittingly identified the problem: since Reception, Caleb had always been seated next to a hearing-impaired child who had now moved to a specialist unit. The teaching assistant who worked with the hearing-impaired child had always explained everything again, generally with simpler language and with lots of images and games to reinforce and consolidate ideas. Caleb had been benefitting from this approach, and had been able to learn and make progress. Without this approach which used visual and kinaesthetic learning, he wasn't able to benefit from teacher talk and didn't understand what was being said. He got through the day by copying what the other children did, but this didn't help him to make progress with his learning.

Caleb's teacher was able to modify her teaching style and put in place a group of peers as 'listening buddies' who Caleb could ask for help and clarification. She taught him memory strategies and before key lessons she made sure that he knew important vocabulary and he had clear outlines of the main points of the lesson. With this support and some 'small steps' targets, Caleb began to make progress again.

Differentiation and inclusion can often appear to be conflicting goals: is it more inclusive to allow a child to do the same activities as the rest of the class, albeit with the support of a teaching assistant, or to differentiate the objective itself to meet the learning needs of the child, even if it means giving them a different activity to complete? The difficulty with the former approach which, on the surface, seems more inclusive, is that it does nothing to address the child's underlying learning difficulties and may contribute to teaching them to be dependent on adult help. It's like jump-starting a car rather than getting a new battery!

Using the *Target Ladders* series will enable non-specialist teachers to identify appropriate learning goals for independent learning, to adapt strategies or ideas listed, and to begin to modify the learning difficulty to close the gap between these children and their peers.

Working memory and auditory processing

Working memory and auditory processing are two separate processes that occur in different parts of the brain. Auditory processing refers to the way in which the auditory nerves in the central nervous system interpret auditory information. The central nervous system is vast and, at a higher level, is also responsible for functions like memory, attention and language. This means that there is a significant overlap in the presentation of Auditory Processing Disorder (APD) and working memory difficulties and the accommodations, interventions and strategies needed to help and support children with the difficulties are often broadly the same. For that reason, it makes sense to develop shared target ladders.

A 'map' showing which part of the brain is involved with which mental process is over-simplistic, because many different brain functions are needed for most processes. However, to help understand working memory and auditory processing we need to know that:

- processes linked to working memory are linked to the prefrontal cortex and parietal lobe;
- sounds are processed in the auditory cortex;
- Broca's area and Wernicke's area are involved in processing receptive and expressive language.

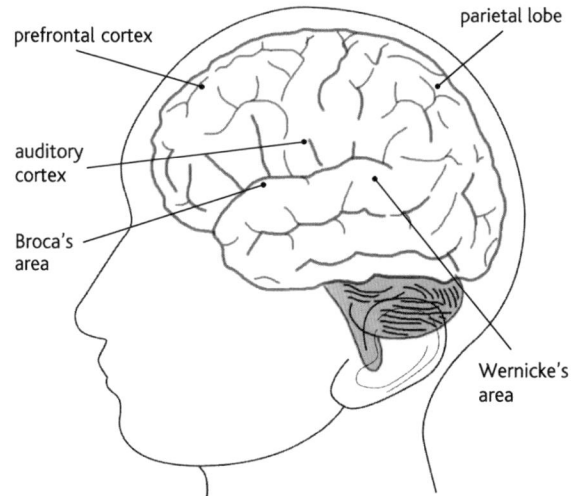

Fig. 1: Simplified diagram showing some parts of the brain involved in working memory and auditory processing.

The prefrontal cortex, just behind the forehead, is where the brain's **central executive** is located. This is where actions are planned based on information taken in by the body's senses (sight, sound, touch, taste, smell, balance and position). **Executive functions** carried out in the prefrontal cortex include:

- attention control: deciding which signals to pay attention to;
- prioritising information received from senses (so a child may prioritise the sound of your voice over the noise of other children's voices);

- learning and concentrating;
- problem solving and decision making;
- distinguishing right from wrong;
- planning movements and activities;
- orchestrating thoughts and actions in accordance with identified goals;
- abstract thinking;
- organising and integrating information;
- flexibility in generating a range of responses;
- self-monitoring and reflecting;
- impulse control and predicting probable outcomes linked to actions;
- social and behavioural regulation;
- managing emotions and showing empathy;
- working memory.

What is working memory?

In *Understanding Working Memory: A Classroom Guide* (Harcourt Assessment, 2007), Gathercole and Alloway, two of the leading researchers into working memory, write:

> Psychologists use the term 'working memory' to describe the ability we have to hold in mind and mentally manipulate information over short periods of time.

Working memory has also been described as the mental equivalent of a sticky note: you make interim jottings on it to store information you need to process, and then discard it once you have processed the information. We need our working memory for all complex mental activities. For example, in order to mentally find $\frac{5}{8}$ of 56, we hold the 5 in our heads while we recall the 8 times table from our long-term memories, divide 56 by 8 to get 7, retrieve the 5, multiply 5 × 7, recall the original sum and say that $\frac{5}{8}$ of 56 = 35.

Working memory is not the same as short-term memory: we use our short-term memory simply to store information for a short time when there is no processing involved. For example, we might use our short-term memory to recall a phone number for the length of time it takes to dial it.

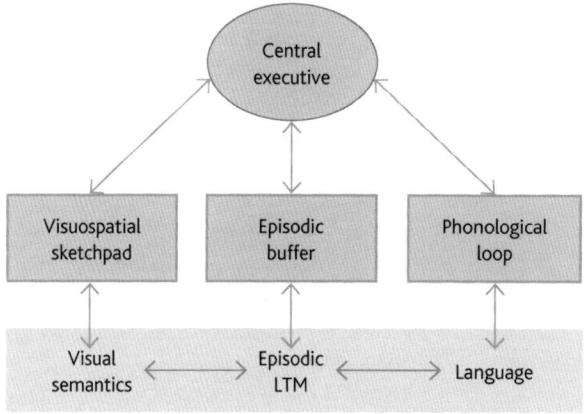

Fig. 2: The multicomponent working memory (Baddeley, 2000).

This model is now standardly used when discussing working memory, and has been confirmed through experimental research to explain the following functions of working memory:

Central executive

The central executive receives visual and auditory information and decides what to pay attention to. So, for example, if you hear two voices, or a voice and a background noise, the central executive allows you to select your focus. It also filters the information received and sends speech-based information into the phonological loop, visual and spatial information into the visuospatial sketchpad and both types of information into the episodic buffer.

The phonological loop

The phonological loop deals with spoken and written information. Short pieces of information (1–2 seconds long) are rehearsed and stored for just long enough to process them. Then they are returned to the central executive, sent to the episodic buffer, sent to the long-term memory or dumped. Within the phonological loop there is a mechanism which converts the written word into a spoken code in order that writing can be processed.

The visuospatial sketchpad

The visuospatial sketchpad deals with visual and spatial information. It allows us to process spatial and visual information and store important ideas in our long-term memory. It can also retrieve information from the long-term memory so, for example, the route to your classroom from the playground will be stored in, and retrievable from, long-term memory once children have walked it a few times.

As we move around, our position in relation to the objects around us changes so we need to be constantly able to update the information on how we relate to our environment. This is achieved partly in the visuospatial sketchpad where the decision as to which information should be stored is made.

The episodic buffer

The episodic buffer combines visual and verbal information and binds information into 'chunks' which can then be stored in, and retrieved from, the long-term memory.

Implications of poor working memory

We use working memory for all aspects of the school curriculum. This list includes some, but by no means all, of the working memory functions for three curriculum activities.

When **reading** we need working memory to:

- remember sound/grapheme correspondences;
- blend words, remembering all of the sounds we've already decoded;
- recognise words on sight when we have only just read them;
- remember which words on the page we've already read so we know which to read next;
- remember all the words in a sentence we're reading so the sentence makes sense;
- remember all the previous sentences we've read so the whole text begins to make sense;

- remember strategies to tackle comprehension questions and perhaps to write the answers.

When **writing** we need working memory to do all of the tasks needed for reading and to:
- remember the overall shape of a text we have already planned;
- remember what we've written so far;
- remember how the current sentence began;
- remember the words already written;
- remember how to spell, or sound out the current word;
- remember how to form, and then to join the letters in the word;
- remember punctuation.

When doing **mental calculations** we need working memory to:
- remember the meaning of each digit and how it relates to other digits;
- remember basic maths facts;
- remember how to perform the different operations;
- remember the numbers we're using in our calculation while we perform the operation;
- remember all the stages in a multi-step problem and keep track of the numbers we generate at each point;
- use estimation to identify the likelihood of our answer being accurate.

Recent studies in America have found that assessment of working memory aged seven years is a much more accurate predictor of attainment at age 11 than any curriculum or other cognitive assessments (www.tracyalloway.com).

What is auditory processing?

Auditory processing is what the brain does with what it hears. APD, also known as Central Auditory Processing Disorder (CAPD), is not a hearing disorder; most children with APD pass hearing tests without difficulty. The ears hear the sounds, but somehow recognition and interpretation of sounds become scrambled in the central nervous system. No one knows why.

Great Ormond Street Hospital (GOSH) states that:

> **Auditory processing disorder (APD) affects how the brain interprets sound rather than how sound is carried through the ear to the brain.**
>
> (GOSH Information sheet on auditory processing, 2014)

The British Society of Audiology in its 2011 *Position Paper on APD* states that APD does not result from failure to understand simple instructions. It lists key characteristics of APD as including:

- poor perception of both speech and non-speech sounds;
- impaired neural function;
- reduced ability to listen, and so to respond appropriately to sounds;
- a collection of symptoms that usually co-occur with other neurodevelopmental disorders.

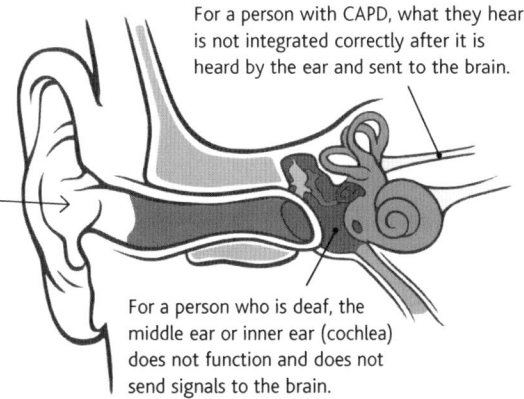

Fig. 3: Diagram showing the location of auditory difficulties.

Listening, which most of us do without thinking, except in noisy situations or when phone reception is bad, is a complex process involving:

- paying attention;
- identifying and discriminating the most important acoustic signal (in a classroom, that should often be the teacher's voice);
- filtering out unnecessary noise;
- recognising each word from its sounds;
- understanding the sentences;
- hearing and interpreting the tone, speed and inflection to enable understanding of the speaker's intention;

- making meaning from what we hear, which frequently involves 'filling the gap' to predict a word we have heard imperfectly;
- making links with what is already known and storing the new information where it will be easily retrieved;
- retrieving information previously stored and comparing it with new information;
- deciding whether to store or dump the new information.

All of these processes and decisions are made without conscious thought and in 'real time'.

It is thought that up to five per cent of children may have some level of APD (Sirimanna & Grant, www.cafamily.org.uk, 2016) where something in the chain of events needed for effective listening is distorted. Each person with APD is affected in a different way and to a different degree, so the difficulties faced by one child with APD may be quite different from those faced by another child. Children with APD tend to experience some degree of interference and distortion in one of more of the following areas:

Auditory figure-ground discrimination

* the ability to identify the most important acoustic signal when there is background noise. Your voice in the classroom may get lost amongst the sounds that most children tune out in a seemingly quiet classroom: the sound of the data projector, the buzzing of fluorescent lights, voices and footsteps in the corridor, the lawn mower outside and the sounds made by the children in class coughing, breathing and fidgeting. All of these sounds are equally prominent for most children with APD.

Auditory discrimination

* the ability to notice, compare and distinguish between distinct and separate sounds, so we recognise similarities and differences in the noises made by the sea and the wind, dropping a pebble and dropping a rock, laughter and sobbing. Auditory discrimination difficulties will also mean that words like *tin* and *pin*, or *like* and *light*, or *power* and *powder* may sound the same.

Auditory memory

* the ability to remember what has been heard, either immediately or later.

Auditory sequencing

* the ability to understand and recall the order of sounds and words. A child might say '*basketti*' instead of '*spaghetti*', or hear the number *318* but write *831* or hear the word *pack* and write *cap*.

Auditory processing speed

* the time taken to perceive the information, to process it and to enact a response. Children with APD are generally much slower than their peers in performing any cognitive task which is language based. When you are giving extended information, they may still be processing your first

sentence when you are beginning the fifth. They then hear the sixth and try to process that, not having heard sentences two, three, four or five. This means that the overall information they receive is incomplete.

Having APD can be equivalent to talking to someone on the phone who is standing in a windy field with reception fading in and out and gusts of wind overpowering the speaker's voice. If you're lucky, you may get some of the message, but it is rarely all of the message and the bits you do hear may be misheard or irrelevant.

Implications of auditory processing difficulties

Because of the difficulties in interpreting the sounds they hear, children with APD frequently experience additional difficulties with some higher order cognitive skills such as:

Expressive language	Children with APD usually have immaturities in their speech for longer than their peers; they take longer to learn to speak in grammatically correct sentences and have a more limited vocabulary.
	Retrieving information is unreliable, often because it has been processed inadequately and stored in one specific location which the child can't access consistently. Even once the information has been retrieved, poor sequencing skills can mean that a word, number or sentence is muddled.
Receptive language	Children with APD often find it hard to understand the meaning of words because they don't make as many categorisations and associations as other children. For example, neurotypical children might classify and mentally store the word *lion* as *African animal*, *meat eater*, *cat family*, *zoo animal*, *medium-sized animal*, *mammal*, *has mane*, *animal that roars*, etc. Any of those associations can be used to retrieve the word *lion*. The child with APD might only classify it under *has mane* so can't recall the word when you do, for example, a project on African animals. The fact that the information retrieval is triggered by a more limited set of ideas helps to explain why a child may seem to know something one day, but not the next.
	The difficulties with processing the auditory signal in the first place means that the language-processing parts of the brain have very little to work with. Comprehension is often incomplete and some basic concepts may be misunderstood. Good comprehension and intact thought processes are needed for most oral problem-solving activities.
Phonological awareness	Phonological awareness enables children to understand the sound structure of words. Children with good phonological awareness can play with rhyme, blend and segment words and think about what makes words the same and different. Poor phonological awareness is a key indicator for dyslexia, but is also present in most children with APD because of the incomplete way in which the auditory signal is processed.

Integration activities	These are activities which require both sides of the brain to work together. Poor integration causes particular issues with curriculum areas such as reading, note-taking, summarising and understanding maths problems as well as hand-eye co-ordination. Children with APD may also have motor and visual processing difficulties. Whereas words are generally processed in the left side of the brain, meaning is often expressed by voice prosodies (pitch, intonation, speed, tone of voice and volume) which are processed on the right side of the brain. The child with APD can't co-ordinate the words with the prosodies and so can't tell from your voice whether you are pleased with them or angry, asking a question or making a statement.
Social skills	Children with APD find it hard to process speech quickly and to participate in faster conversations. For younger children, social skills are mostly mediated through action, with speech providing a narrative, so children with APD may well play with their peers. However, by the time they are eight or nine years old language becomes more important in negotiating friendships and social groupings. A child who can't follow a fast conversation can easily become socially isolated.
Attention and concentration	When the auditory signal is distorted and processing is slow, it's hard to pay attention; if you haven't fully understood the information or the instructions to complete a task, interest, concentration and motivation may be limited.
Behaviour	Children who sit in the classroom feeling as if it is not relevant to them will often display unwanted behaviours due to frustration, low self-esteem, boredom or to distract attention from learning difficulties and focus it on behaviour instead.
Working memory	Since the processing of any information takes longer, more of the auditory message is lost from working memory. This means that the information which is eventually processed and stored may bear little relationship to the speaker's intended message.

Working memory difficulties, APD and other specific learning difficulties

Working memory difficulties and APD are specific learning difficulties since they are not linked to intelligence and don't necessarily impact on the child's entire curriculum attainment; children with working memory difficulties and/or APD may be skilled at non-language-based tasks like art, PE, music or activities which don't depend on quick retrieval of information.

It is common to find working memory difficulties and APD with other specific learning difficulties like Attention Deficit Disorder (ADD), Attention Deficit Hyperactivity Disorder (ADHD), dyslexia, specific language impairment (SLI) and autism. Bear in mind, however, that not all learning difficulties are linked to working memory or APD, and that not all primary-school-aged children with working memory difficulties or APD will exhibit learning difficulties; some learn effective coping strategies from an early age.

All of the learning difficulties most commonly associated with working memory and auditory processing involve cognitively higher order processes, primarily language.

AD(H)D

There are so many difficulties that children with AD(H)D and APD have in common that many children with APD are initially diagnosed as having AD(H)D and some children have both APD and AD(H)D. Working memory is a continual battle for children with AD(H)D because there is always a question over whether the difficulty is with their attention, or their memory. Key indicators of AD(H)D include inattention, distractibility and difficulties with understanding or remembering verbal information. These are all seen in children who experience working memory difficulties and APD as well. The key difference in behaviour is that the child with working memory difficulties or APD can generally sit and focus in a quiet space, if you can find a space that is quiet enough, whereas the child with AD(H)D is inattentive and distractible in all contexts. Also, AD(H)D medication won't help a child with working memory difficulties or APD.

In spite of the behavioural similarities, the underlying causes of the conditions are different. For children with AD(H)D, the difficulty with paying attention disrupts learning; children with working memory difficulties forget what they have been told; and children with APD lose attention only because they can't process the verbal information.

Specific language impairment (SLI)

In the absence of any other neurodevelopmental difficulty, children who have more difficulty than their peers in acquiring language may be diagnosed with having a specific language impairment. Some children diagnosed with SLI may well have an underlying working memory difficulty or perceptual difficulty such as APD. In many cases, the difference between a diagnosis of SLI and one of APD depends on the child's ability to process non-speech sounds.

Children with SLI generally have unimpaired auditory processing. For them the signals are scrambled at a much higher-order level in the brain. The difference between SLI and APD has been described as the difference between listening to the poem 'Jabberwocky' and playing Chinese whispers. A child with SLI may hear, process and identify every syllable and word perfectly clearly, but the meaning is jumbled and many of the words don't make sense; a child playing Chinese whispers often ends up with a message which is only partially heard and which no longer makes sense because it's not the original message intended by the speaker. The child with working memory difficulties may have either forgotten what they were told in the first place, or they didn't pay attention because they had no confidence in their ability to recall the information.

The outcome for each set of children is that their language acquisition is slow and they have difficulties making sense of what they hear and in information retrieval.

Dyslexia

The three major indicators of dyslexia are poor working memory, slow processing speed and poor phonological awareness, so the comorbidity of dyslexia, working memory difficulties and APD is very common. Without a good working memory, it will always be difficult to demonstrate good phonological awareness.

Some people regard dyslexia as primarily a language disorder, rather than specifically a literacy one: literacy being regarded as one facet of language processing. Children with dyslexia often have limited receptive or expressive spoken language as well as difficulties with written language. Being very dyslexic has been described as like being surrounded by people who speak a foreign language with which you have enough familiarity to understand only the gist of what is being said, and to make only the gist of your meaning understood. Many children with language processing difficulties are unable to access the full detail and the gentle nuances in tone and meaning of a conversation or text.

Autism

Autistic Spectrum Condition (ASC) is another neurodevelopmental difficulty which shares many diagnostic features with working memory difficulties and APD. Most children with autism have poor working memory and the majority have difficulties with some aspects of language use. Children with autism experience difficulties with integration (where both sides of the brain work together) which lead to curriculum challenges as well as social challenges. Although we generally process words and sentences in the left hemisphere of the brain, speech prosodies (tone of voice, etc.) are processed in the right hemisphere. Poor integration explains why many children with autism find it hard to know whether you're being happy, cross, tired, sarcastic or ironic and this can lead to social friction. Like children with APD, those with autism find non-literal meanings, particularly idioms, metaphors and similes, hard to follow.

Although some children with high-functioning autism have good visuospatial working memory, the majority of all children with autism have poor verbal working memory. Children with autism also find it hard to shift their focus from one activity to another because their central executive (see Baddeley's working memory diagram on page 10) finds it hard to shift the focus and reprioritise tasks to identify a different activity. Not knowing what to focus on can mimic behaviours of inattention that are frequently associated with working memory difficulties and APD as well as the conduct behaviours linked to frustration, low self-esteem, boredom or to distract attention from learning difficulties and focus it on behaviour instead.

Diagnosis

Deciding whether to seek a diagnosis is always a difficult decision for a family. Some children and families are relieved if they receive a diagnosis because they feel it offers an explanation for the difficulties the child faces; other children and parents dislike being 'labelled' and so resist diagnosis. The decision is very personal. A diagnosis doesn't change or alleviate the difficulties the child faces, but it can be helpful in indicating ways of supporting them. However, the same targets and activities can be used to support a child whether or not any diagnosis has been sought or given.

Diagnosing working memory difficulties

A diagnosis of working memory difficulties can only be made by an educational psychologist or a paediatrician. The diagnosis will only be made if working memory is weak and there are no other associated neurodevelopmental difficulties.

It is unlikely that an educational psychologist would wish to make a diagnosis of working memory difficulties in children under the age of seven years old because variability in hearing, language development, the child's maturity and their experience can impact so significantly on their ability to listen and learn. The impact of working memory difficulties also becomes increasingly apparent in children of 7+ as the curriculum becomes more language based, fewer visual cues are used and there is greater expectation that a child should pay attention and concentrate for longer periods. Children are also increasingly expected to process extended chunks of language, recall and retrieve information swiftly and be able to do mental arithmetic, read, write and spell.

There are some classroom assessments that can give you an indication about working memory difficulties. One easily available assessment is the Digit Memory Test by Turner and Rissdale (see 'digits test' at www.dyslexia-international.org). The standardisation for this test is not reliable, but it will give you an indication of how many items a child can remember and repeat (short-term memory) and how many they can process to repeat in reverse order (working memory). If you look online, you will find other indicative tests of a similar sort.

The most useful guide of a child's working memory difficulties will be through observation. Pearson (www.pearsonclinical.co.uk) publishes the Working Memory Rating Scale (WMRS) which is an observation-based checklist which draws attention to memory issues children find taxing. Pearson also publishes the Automated Working Memory Assessment (AWMA) which is a comprehensive, computer-based working memory assessment.

The checklist on pages 21–23 can be used to highlight areas of concern. An educational psychologist will probably be interested to see what you have identified, but will do a battery of other tests to exclude other developmental difficulties and to explain working memory expectations for typically-developing children of the same age as the child about whom you have concerns.

Diagnosing APD

As with working memory APD is rarely diagnosed in children under the age of seven years old because variability in hearing, language development, the child's maturity and their experience can impact so significantly on their ability to listen and learn. The impact of APD becomes increasingly apparent in children of 7+ as the curriculum becomes more language based, fewer visual cues are used and there is greater expectation that a child should pay attention and concentrate for longer periods. Children are also expected to process extended chunks of language, recall and retrieve information swiftly and be able to do mental arithmetic, read, write and spell.

Although checklists (such as the one on pages 21–23) are useful in identifying the difficulties that children face in school, they cannot be used to diagnose APD. The route to diagnosis, depending on where you live, will normally be:

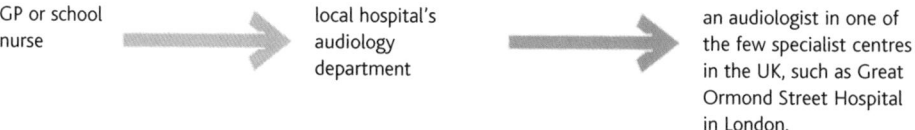

GP or school nurse → local hospital's audiology department → an audiologist in one of the few specialist centres in the UK, such as Great Ormond Street Hospital in London.

Before reaching the specialist audiologist, the referral process initiated by the school will generally involve: the class teacher – to comment on the child's academic performance and behaviour in school (and here the checklists can be invaluable); a speech therapist – who will generally be asked to assess the child's speech and language towards the beginning of the referral process; and an educational psychologist – who can shed light on overall cognitive function in different areas. This is generally sought by the school early in the assessment process.

If a referral to a specialist audiologist is deemed appropriate, they will evaluate the information gained from these professionals and administer a series of highly specialised tests in a sound-proof room. Only an audiologist can make a firm diagnosis of APD.

Identifying children with working memory difficulties or APD in your classroom

Whilst some children with working memory difficulties or APD will gain a diagnosis, many others won't but will still need to have their learning needs met. Children with APD or poor working memory will struggle to learn at the same rate their peers do because so many of the building blocks of successful classroom learning are dependent on accurate listening and working memory.

Although having an identified diagnosis may bring benefits, for the class teacher the imperative is to educate the individual child through Quality First Teaching (QFT), differentiation, reasonable adjustments and putting in place relevant evidence-based interventions. In order to do this, it is useful to know what a child can do in order to build on strengths and address barriers to learning.

Working memory difficulties and APD indicators

The following list represents a consensus about some of the behaviours shown by children with working memory difficulties and APD but is not intended to be used as an assessment tool. Instead it is a reminder of the range of needs experienced by children with working memory difficulties and APD. Most aspects of working memory difficulties and APD will have implications for a child's performance and attainment across the taught curriculum, and in addition, for behaviour.

Although the list is not intended to be used as a screening tool, if you teach a child for whom you answer 'Yes' *when compared to the majority of children of the same age* to most of the questions, and the difficulties are severe and persistent, it would be wise to seek further advice from an expert. You are very unlikely to tick all of the boxes for any child. The behaviours for which there is no tick in either column are sometimes observed in children with APD or working memory difficulties but may also be indicative of other neurodevelopmental difficulties and may be of interest to psychologists or doctors.

	APD	Working memory	CHILD
Concentration, attention, understanding			
Easily distracted	✓	✓	
Short attention span for a self-chosen activity			
Short attention span for an adult-chosen activity	✓	✓	
Short attention span in whole-class listening time	✓	✓	
Attention is inconsistent	✓		
Restless/bored/disruptive in whole-class listening time	✓	✓	
Easily distracted by background noise	✓		
Difficulties in dividing attention (e.g. between teacher voice and current activity)	✓	✓	
Trouble making links between what is already known and new ideas	✓	✓	
Learning behaviours			
Easily frustrated	✓	✓	
Gives up quickly when the task is challenging	✓	✓	
Learns by seeing and doing, not by being told	✓	✓	
Struggles with the logical thought processes needed to solve problems	✓	✓	
Appears to be 'in their own little world'/daydreams	✓	✓	
Can't cope with mistakes or imperfections in a piece of work			
Self-assessment is unreliable and variable	✓	✓	
Watches instead of/before joining in with group activities	✓	✓	
Low self-esteem	✓	✓	
Impulsive – struggles with self-regulation			
Finds transitions from activity to activity hard	✓		
Struggles to settle to a new activity	✓	✓	
Has social difficulties	✓		
Poor emotional literacy	✓		
Either withdrawn or the 'class clown'	✓	✓	

Working Memory and Auditory Processing

	APD	Working memory	CHILD
Memory			
Needs help/reminding to follow three-step instructions	✓	✓	
Has incomplete recall of what is said	✓	✓	
Forgets what was said within a few minutes	✓	✓	
Forgets what was said yesterday/last week/last month	✓	✓	
Can't summarise or identify the main idea of teacher talk	✓	✓	
Forgets what they seemed to know before	✓	✓	
Benefits from routines, rules and consistency	✓	✓	
Does not remember classroom routines	✓	✓	
Forgets the sequence of ideas/instructions	✓	✓	
Ideas are often disorganised	✓	✓	
Forgets what needs to be done and abandons the task	✓	✓	
Disorganised/forgetful	✓	✓	
Listening and language			
Had/has/needed/needs speech and language therapy	✓	✓	
Needs additional 'take-up-time' to process information and answer questions	✓	✓	
Overreacts to loud noises	✓		
Misunderstands what is said/says '*Pardon?/What?/Huh?*' frequently	✓	✓	
Difficulty understanding implications of speech prosodies and non-literal meaning	✓		
Difficulty in following and contributing to conversations	✓	✓	
Slow to respond in conversation	✓	✓	
Receptive vocabulary is limited and conceptual development immature	✓	✓	
Expressive vocabulary is limited and sentence structures are simple and immature	✓	✓	
Needs to be reminded several times to stop and listen	✓		
Uses a lot of non-specific language (e.g. '*thingy*') and generalised adjectives (e.g. '*big*', '*little*', '*nice*')	✓	✓	
Answers questions with irrelevant information	✓		
Can't link what is seen to what is heard	✓		
Literacy			
Poor phonological awareness	✓	✓	
Slow to learn sound/symbol relationships	✓	✓	
Difficulty in identifying/generating rhyming words	✓	✓	
Difficulty in discriminating between words/sounds	✓		
Slow to blend sounds to make words	✓	✓	
Limited repertoire of sight vocabulary	✓	✓	
Decodes, but doesn't understand	✓	✓	
Pace of reading is slow and hesitant	✓	✓	
Loses their place when reading	✓	✓	
Knows a word on one page but not the next	✓	✓	
Over-reliant on pictures when reading	✓	✓	

	APD	Working memory	CHILD
Slow progress in reading/writing/spelling	✓	✓	
Poor spelling	✓	✓	
Untidy handwriting		✓	
Limited range of sentence structures in writing	✓	✓	
Texts are not well organised		✓	
Orally good, but disappointing recorded work		✓	
Struggles to copy from the board		✓	
Engages in displacement activities in order to delay starting a piece of literacy work	✓	✓	
Maths			
Slow to learn to relate quantity to numerals		✓	
Finds it hard to learn language for maths	✓	✓	
Finds maths problems hard	✓	✓	
Performance is inconsistent	✓	✓	
Finds it hard to learn and retain number facts	✓	✓	
Difficulty learning the concept of time	✓	✓	
Place-keeping errors – loses the thread during mental arithmetic	✓	✓	

Creating a working memory- and APD-friendly classroom

> *If a child can't learn the way we teach, maybe we should teach the way they learn.*
>
> Ignacio Estrada

A classroom that supports children with working memory difficulties and APD will support all children, since all children will benefit from the strategies you put in place. The following list is divided into sections containing ideas for different aspects of teaching and learning. Different suggestions will be appropriate for different age-groups and children. Some of these ideas will be appropriate for your situation while there will be good reasons why others are not suitable for you. You are probably doing much of what the list suggests anyway, because many of these ideas represent quality first teaching. Take from this list only what is relevant for the learners in your classroom and for you.

General advice

- Offer structured, 'small steps' teaching with overlearning built in.
- Make learning active, with positive feedback and focused praise.
- 'Show', don't just 'tell', and whenever possible give opportunities for the children to 'do'.
- Make maximum use of ICT, including interactive whiteboards, PCs, laptops and tablets.
- Create a multi-sensory teaching environment. Use images, diagrams, flow charts, colours, mind maps, sounds and tactile objects. Each of these sensory opportunities allows the children to make memories which support what they have heard and been taught.
- Include active, problem-solving approaches.
- Give clear indicators of time left in an activity.
- Be patient and prepared to repeat yourself several times.
- As far as possible, ensure that the classroom is peaceful and free from distractions.
- Allow full access to the subjects the child is good at.
- Ensure that all children have easy access to pencils, erasers and so on. Children with APD and working memory difficulties don't have capacity to worry about these small practical things alongside the bigger task of listening and engaging.
- Avoid lengthy demonstration and explanations.

- Break down instructions and long sections of teacher talk into chunks.
- Use 'think, pair, share' of key ideas to give children time to process what they've heard and rephrase it to a partner before sharing with the class.

Supporting children who have working memory difficulties

Gathercole and Alloway (*Working Memory and Learning: A Practical Guide for Teachers*, SAGE Publications, 2008) recommend the following strategies:

Principle	Further information
Recognise working memory failures	Warning signs include incomplete recall, failure to follow instructions, place-keeping errors and task abandonment
Monitor the child	Look out for warning signs and ask the child what they think they should do next
Evaluate working memory load when necessary	Heavy loads can be caused by lengthy sequences, unfamiliar and meaningless content and demanding mental-processing activities
Reduce working memory loads when necessary	Reduce the amount of material to be remembered, increase the meaningfulness and familiarity of the material, simplify mental processing and restructure complex tasks
Repeat important information	Repetition can be supplied by teachers or fellow pupils nominated as memory guides
Encourage use of memory aids	These include wall charts and posters, useful spellings, personalised dictionaries, cubes, counters, abaci, number lines, multiplication grids, calculators, memory cards, audio recorders and computer software
Develop the child's own strategies to support memory	These include asking for help, rehearsal, note-taking, use of long-term memory, place-keeping and organisational strategies

Interventions and strategies for improving working memory

There is continuing debate about whether interventions to improve working memory are effective. Children generally improve at the activities they practice during the intervention, but the transfer of strategies into the classroom and their longer-term impact on learning is less clear. Research is increasingly focused on electronic memory interventions such as:

- Cogmed (www.pearsonclinical.co.uk/Cogmed);
- Jungle Memory™ (www.junglememory.com);
- Mastering Memory (www.masteringmemory.co.uk);
- FastForWord® (www.scilearnglobal.com);
- Cellfield (www.cellfielduk.com).

These interventions are all based on work by, and are sometimes developed by, well-respected researchers. The interventions are therefore evidence based and it is easy to find research articles and reviews online. However, none of these are cheap to buy and each approach will benefit children with particular learning difficulties, learning styles and interests. There is no 'one size fits all' intervention. Some interventions offer a free trial or demonstration. There is also a wide range of non-electronic memory activities, games and interventions which are intended for use by children between about the ages of 3–12 years. These are widely used in schools and many report good outcomes from using them.

No matter which kind of intervention children experience, the strategies developed by the interventions are often ones that use children's learning strengths and that can be taught and practised throughout the school day. The strategies will need to be modelled constantly and supported if children are to turn to them independently. They include:

Rehearsal

This is a very useful strategy, particularly when information needs to be held in short-term memory for a short time. Rehearsal involves keeping information within the phonological loop (see working memory diagram on page 10). As children mature, the number of digits, words and sentences they can hold in their short-term memory (simply holding and reciting the information) as well as in their working memory (processing the information) increases. The progression given below is indicative only since different studies show different results.

Approximate age (years)	Number of digits held in short-term memory	Number of digits held in working memory
4–5	3	–
5–6	4	2
6–7	5	3
8–10	6	4
10–12	6–7	5

Table 1 shows the indicative age at which typically-developing children can hold digits in their short-term and working memory, based on findings from a range of research studies.

Rehearsal can also be useful as a working memory strategy as children learn to 'dual track'. (For example, if you had to say your postcode backwards, you would probably have to repeat at least parts of it forwards while you simultaneously said aloud the numbers and letters in the required order.)

Rehearsal is the strategy that children use most often, even though it is limited and, as soon as any distraction intervenes, the information slips from the phonological loop and cannot then be retrieved.

Visualisation

If children have a stronger visual memory than auditory memory, they may find visualising the information to be recalled – by capturing a mental photograph and seeing it in the 'mind's eye' – a useful strategy.

Visualisation is useful for mental maths if children have experienced making images of number facts or problems. Children talk about mentally 'parking' numbers in certain places until they are needed and this can be a particularly useful strategy for securing spelling and phonics.

Visualisation is particularly useful if the activity involves remembering patterns or activities that rely on spatial awareness. Be aware, however, that some children experience aphantasia – an inability to visualise or to make visual memories – and for these children visualisation is not a useful technique.

Storytelling/picturing

It can take children a while to learn this strategy but it's very effective if used properly. The aim is to tell yourself a short story, based on familiar places or routes, which includes the items to be remembered in that familiar setting. (So, for example, to remember the list: *cow, calculator, photo* and *tree* the 'story' might be: *A cow came into the reception area of our school and asked how much she had to pay for school milk. Miss Webb got out her calculator and showed the cow. The cow took a photo of the number on her phone, then wandered off and sat under a tree in front of the school.*)

Storytelling usually has to be modelled several times, with the child being asked about where they think the objects should be placed. The funnier the story the better because humour helps to make memories too.

Before asking the child to list the objects, make sure that you and they have told the story aloud.

Making notes and graphic organisers

Notes don't have to be words; they can equally well be numbers or little sketch images. Encourage the child to try making notes in different formats so they learn what works for them. Teach children to identify key information in a mental maths question and to jot down the numbers they need to manipulate. Help them to use mind maps and word webs and other graphic organisers so they have a choice of ways of recording information. The more often you model the use of these organisational tools, the more likely children will use them independently.

Teaching someone else

Teaching is an excellent mechanism for exploring your own understanding and checking that you remember and include the key information.

Movement

For some children, movement is the best way of storing and recalling information. It may be the movement involved with physically placing a coloured sticky note with information on it in a particular place; or the movement associated with actions, for example, skipping to the three times table and hopping to the four times table; or the muscle-memory we form when we repeat an action over and over again, so, for example, recalling letter formation, or learning how to do a forward roll.

These are the strategies most commonly recommended. However, if a child is to learn to make purposeful use of these strategies, they need to be explicitly reminded to use them throughout the day at school. In this way, they learn when and why it is appropriate to use one strategy instead of another and their use of the strategy becomes more intuitive.

Additional ideas and strategies include:

Pre-teaching and post-tutoring	Before you teach a lesson, work with a small group of children to check that concepts that you plan to build on are established and understood. Where possible and appropriate, allow them to see, feel, touch and do reinforcement activities. These shouldn't be worksheets. Check vocabulary is understood and can be used correctly. Introduce key new ideas for the lesson, together with vocabulary, through: • practical work with tactile objects to explore basic concepts; • paper-based activities like matching vocabulary to definitions; making mind maps and word grids to record what is already known; • talking tasks – chatting around the subject; • research tasks – going online or finding and talking about books which give insights into the subject area. After a lesson has been taught, work with the pre-teaching group to: • check learning of key ideas and concepts; • confirm and embed vocabulary; • practise any homework activities to reinforce vocabulary and concepts.
Magpie competitions	Activate prior knowledge or develop vocabulary banks for writing by inviting children to share ideas. • Draw a grid on a piece of paper. (The grid is particularly important for boys, who often like boxes!) • Label the boxes. These could be alphabetical (which might be grouped *a–d*, *e–h*, etc.), headings (e.g. adjectives, adverbs, verbs or clothes, food, houses, etc.) or labelled in any other way to enable children to organise the information they are retrieving. • Challenge children to write at least one word in each of the boxes in 3 minutes. • At the end of 3 minutes, ask children to compare their words with at least five other people, more if possible. Tell children that if another child has a word they don't have, the other child gets a point and they write down the word (and vice versa). • At the end of 5 minutes, find out who had most points. Note that all of the children now have much fuller sheets of paper and they have been talking about the subject for 8 minutes before you start the lesson.
True and false	Prepare a list of statements which are linked to the topic of the lesson. (The number of statements can vary according to the age and stage of your class). One or more of the statements should be untrue. Use key facts for your true statements, and obscure non-facts for the others. • Begin the lesson by handing out the list of statements. • Tell the children that at least one, and maybe more, of the statements is false. • Ask children to work in pairs to discuss the statements and decide which are true. Now, when you begin your lesson, all of the children are pre-warned about key points you want them to remember, they have discussed the main ideas and they will listen as you talk, to try to spot information relating to the statements. • After the lesson, ask children to revisit the statements and check whether or not they made the right choices. You can differentiate this activity by having some children read more, or longer, statements.
Mind maps	Teach children how to make and read mind maps to record summaries of information and to show how different ideas are linked. • Before the lesson, hand out incomplete mind maps. The gaps can be for drawing, writing one or two words or note-making, depending on the age and stage of your children. The mind maps should show the main themes and ideas of this lesson, possibly linked to prior knowledge. • Let the children complete the mind maps as you talk. This activity structures the information in a way that provides a model showing how information is related as well as drawing the children's attention to key information from this and previous lessons. You can differentiate the activity by the complexity of the mind maps and the amount of information you complete.

Supporting children who have APD

All of the strategies provided for children who experience working memory difficulties will also support children with APD, however children with APD will also benefit from these additional strategies.

Children with APD need a classroom environment in which background noise is minimised. They will benefit from:

- the best possible classroom acoustics (e.g. carpets on the floor, window blinds, drapes on display tables to minimise hard surfaces, etc.);
- a soundfield system to support and ensure that there is clear sound throughout your classroom;
- a 'volume control' visual which you can point at to show children where the classroom noise is and where it needs to be for a given session;
- sitting close to you so that you can check discreetly if they have understood and you can pick up on non-verbal communication if they're struggling. Make sure they are not near doors and windows which might offer distractions;
- seeing your face and mouth: ensure you are standing with a light source on your face, and not behind you;
- all children knowing that whispering, playing with Velcro™, etc. is unacceptable during listening times.

Children with APD need listening support. They will benefit from:

- repetition or rephrasing of key information throughout the lesson;
- key words being written clearly (if the child can read);
- the use of colour and space for key words so that even a child who can't read can use visuospatial information to remember the words;
- having a signal to alert the child that a key point is being made;
- using images and gestures as you speak; many children with APD learn to link your gestures to the key facts;
- a quiet area or privacy screen for independent work;
- carefully chosen partners and groupings for paired and group work;
- task charts (see page 63); as you repeat your instructions for the child, quickly sketch little images. The quality of the artwork doesn't matter: the intention is to provide a visual prompt for the instruction.

Sound therapies

A number of different types of commercial therapeutic interventions are available, all of which claim to help some people with APD. Whilst we cannot recommend, or vouch for, any of them you may want to explore some of the better researched sound therapies like:

- The Listening Programme® (www.learning-solutions.co.uk);
- Johansen Individualised Auditory Stimulation (www.dyslexia-lab.dk; info@johansensoundtherapy.com);
- The Tomatis® Method (www.tomatis.com; www.tuneyourears.com).

At the time of publication, all of these programmes are available in the UK – centres tend to be distributed around the UK. Some of the programmes are exclusive to APD, but most claim to help children with other associated neurodevelopmental conditions such as autism or ADHD or learning difficulties such as dyslexia.

Supporting children who have attention difficulties

The most important strategy is to demystify the issue: help children to understand what attention is and what it feels like to focus on something, even for a short time. Help children to know what their strengths are while you use an intervention to teach them strategies for paying attention.

- **Fidget toys** can be helpful. Children with attention difficulties often need to use their bodies at the same time as they use their minds. If they are concentrating on staying still, they aren't concentrating on what you are saying. Fidget toys can help children to focus, absorb more information, self-regulate and calm down. Establish clear rules for the use of fidget toys but don't make them a battleground and don't give them as rewards. If a child needs a fidget toy, they should routinely have access to it. There are many fidget toys available; you need to find out which type will work for an individual learner. Some children prefer a thick rubber band or piece of sticky-tak which doesn't draw attention to them.
- **Weighted items on the shoulder, back or lap.** There is a wide range of toys, blankets, vests and backpacks which are often filled with wheat or gel and which some children find soothing. You can try out the principle by placing a therapeutic wheat bag (gently heated or unheated) around the shoulders or in the lap of an inattentive child, or by putting a heavy catalogue in a backpack. When weighted items work, they reduce anxiety and stress, ease irritability and restlessness, help with self-regulation and improve focus.
- **Sensory breaks.** Create opportunities for the child to have short breaks during which they can move. Some children benefit from a 'sensory break' card which they can show to you before going to a designated place in or near the classroom and engaging in a brief, movement-based activity. If you use Time Out as a punishment, ensure that these breaks are called movement or sensory breaks to recognise that they are therapeutic, not punitive.
- **Use gesture.** Agree gestures or signals that you can use discretely to refocus the attention of a distracted child. A gentle shoulder tap or placing your hand on their table may be enough.
- **Call attention to key information.** Evolve a phrase like *'Listen carefully now,'* which will signal to all children and specifically those who are distractible that this is important information.
- **Keep curriculum talk and management talk** as separate as possible. A child who is struggling to listen and follow will find it particularly hard to distinguish between what you are saying about the topic, and when you're giving class management instructions to children (e.g. *'The hole in the top of the volcano is called the crater. Kieron can you open the window for me? The lava comes up the vent and ...'*).

- **Discourage frenetic work patterns.** In order to discourage a child from dashing off something in order to be first finished, make thought and presentation part of the success criteria for a piece of work. Try to avoid phrases like '*As soon as you've finished, you can go out to play.*'

Supporting children who have poor language development

It is widely acknowledged that oral language is critical for literacy development and academic success. Most children with working memory difficulties or APD will have poor language development. Very often, this also means that their conceptual development and their ability to link and classify words is poorly developed.

Dr Marion Blank, a well-known developmental psychologist, devised language levels to show how children's language development moves from answering direct questions to understanding abstract ideas. Blank's levels can be used to support children who show developmental delay in language skills and describe language development up to the point that a typically developing child reaches at about 6–7 years old. They are, however, very helpful in identifying missing concepts and language targets for older children. You can find resources to support Blank's language levels on the TES website (www.tes.com/teaching-resources) and on the ELKLAN website (www.elklan.co.uk) as well as other website that support the development of language.

Once you have identified what the child can do securely and what their difficulties are, you can apply more focused interventions to support them. Always be guided by the stage the child is working at, not the grammar curriculum.

- **Vocabulary**: move from concrete to abstract. Make lists of 'core' and 'challenge' words which children need to know or to learn during a curriculum focus (e.g. a geography unit on coastal areas might assume children know a core vocabulary like *sea, sand, deep, beach, cliff, rock, seaweed, boat, ship,* but they may also need to learn challenge words such as *coast, ocean, shallow, tide, pebble, rock pool, tanker, yacht*). Don't make assumptions about what they know: check which words the child consistently knows using different pictures and contexts and teach the rest using pictures and multi-media.
- **Word endings**: ensure the child knows, hears and uses noun and verb inflections like *-s, -ing, -ed*. Do children know when to use them and what they mean? Are they able to use irregular forms of plurals (e.g. *mice, children*) and past tenses (e.g. *went, caught*)?
- **Function words**: nouns and verbs are easier to learn and use than determiners such as *the, this, these, that, those, a* and *an*. Make sure the child knows when to use these words. Also, ensure that their use of pronouns is accurate and enables you to follow what the child is talking about.
- **Sentence structure**: use writing mats and coloured shapes to show how nouns, verbs and other words are organised into simple sentences. Once the child is securely using simple sentences, use tactile and multi-media resources to secure compound and complex sentences.

Supporting children who have social difficulties

Children with working memory difficulties and APD are often socially isolated at school. The Department for Education's 2014 publication *Mental Health and Behaviour in Schools* acknowledges that 1 in 10 of children aged between five and 16 years old has a clinically diagnosable mental health disorder and about 1 in 7 has a less severe difficulty. The report states that primary schools must aim **"to identify and address those with less severe needs at an early stage and build their resilience."** The report recognises that many potential mental health difficulties can be prevented, or at least mitigated, by building resilience which has several inter-related elements:

> Firstly, a sense of self-esteem and confidence; secondly a belief in one's own self-efficacy and ability to deal with change and adaptation; and thirdly a repertoire of social problem solving approaches.
>
> *(Mental Health and Behaviour in Schools*, DfE, 2014)

The recommendation in *Mental Health and Behaviour in Schools* is that schools should use Goodman's Strengths and Difficulties Questionnaire (www.sdqinfo.org) in order to assess difficulties, identify children for an intervention and then evaluate the impact.

The aim should be for you to take a targeted approach to promoting mental health in which:

- **all** children have weekly PSHE sessions which focus on specific strategies and contexts;
- **some** children have social skills interventions, supporting and augmenting the work with the whole class;
- **few** children access one-to-one counselling, play therapy or Child and Adolescent Mental Health Services (CAMHS) to address their more significant social, emotional and mental health (SEMH) difficulties.

The aim of a social skills intervention should be primarily to focus on building resilience through encouraging *self-esteem and confidence using strategies to develop self-efficacy and ability to deal with change through a repertoire of social problem solving approaches.*

Children with working memory difficulties and APD are likely to struggle if your intervention is very focused on listening. Instead, try an intervention which involves role-play, games and activities. Role-play, in particular, is very powerful and allows you to develop 'scripts' for children to use in commonly encountered social scenarios.

A wide range of social skills approaches and interventions are widely available such as *Time to Talk*, *Socially Speaking* and *The Friendship Formula* (all available from LDA). It is always important to match the intervention to the child's needs, not the child to whichever intervention you happen to have available.

How to use this book

You will find a simple four-step summary of how to use this book on page 36.

Every child with working memory and auditory processing difficulties has different strengths and weaknesses. The priority for addressing these will be determined by the difficulties currently being faced by the child and will depend on your professional judgement, supported by the child's current anxieties.

To support you with focused target setting, the book is structured as follows:

- Seven different Aspects of working memory and auditory processing difficulties have been identified (see Fig. 4 on page 34). Think about the child's difficulties: which of these Aspects is causing most concern at the moment?
- Within each Aspect there are four different Target Ladders, each based on a particular area of challenge. This is intended to help you to think carefully about precisely where the barrier may be.
- The relevant Target Ladder can then be used to identify the 'next step' target for the child.
- Suggested activities and strategies offer classroom-friendly ideas so you can support the child to meet their target.

For example, as you can see in Fig. 5 on page 35, difficulties with **Aspect 3: Auditory processing for communication** can be subdivided into specific areas to work on: receptive language, expressive language, semantics and pragmatics and social communication. Each Target Ladder contains 24 targets.

Aspects, Target Ladders and targets

Aspects

The seven different Aspects identified in this book describe contexts and difficulties which are frequently faced by children who have working memory or auditory processing difficulties. In order to identify the most appropriate Aspect for a particular child, you will need to consider the most significant barrier for the child: for example, is it that the child is unable to remember common maths facts or that they struggle to hear the sounds in a word?

The Aspects of working memory and auditory processing difficulties identified in this book are:

1 Auditory processing and exploring sound
2 Auditory processing for phonological development
3 Auditory processing for communication
4 Auditory memory
5 Visual-spatial memory
6 Kinasthetic memory
7 Memory, attention and organisation

Target Ladders

Each of the Aspects is further subdivided into four Target Ladders, each of which addresses different parts of the Aspect. These enable you to develop your understanding of the child's individual needs, 'drilling down' to assist you to identify the child's particular strengths and weaknesses. The Target Ladders are set out on pages 42–83.

SEN	7 Aspects	28 Target Ladders	Targets
Working memory and auditory processing difficulties	1 Auditory processing and exploring sound	Pitch and volume Beat, rhythm, location Making sounds Background noise	24 targets 24 targets 24 targets 24 targets
	2 Auditory processing for phonological development	Identifying sounds Speech sounds Blending sounds Rhyme	24 targets 24 targets 24 targets 24 targets
	3 Auditory processing for communication	Receptive Language Expressive language Semantics and pragmatics Social communication	24 targets 24 targets 24 targets 24 targets
	4 Auditory memory	Recall Listening and remembering Instruction processing Sequencing	24 targets 24 targets 24 targets 24 targets
	5 Visual-spatial memory	Matching and remembering objects Matching and remembering shapes and symbols Matching and remembering location Matching and remembering patterns	24 targets 24 targets 24 targets 24 targets
	6 Kinasthetic memory	Copying movements Copying symbols Hand–eye co-ordination Handwriting	24 targets 24 targets 24 targets 24 targets
	7 Memory, attention and organisation	Attention Planning Organisation Prioritising	24 targets 24 targets 24 targets 24 targets

Fig. 4: The structure of *Target Ladders: working memory and auditory processing*.

Targets

There are 24 targets in each Target Ladder, with the simplest ones labelled with the letter A, then moving through the alphabet up to L, which are the most difficult. In each Target Ladder there are two rows that are labelled with the same letter, because all of the targets in those rows are at a similar developmental level. It is unlikely that any child will need to have all of the targets in each letter band: use your knowledge of the child to identify what they already know and to prioritise what is important.

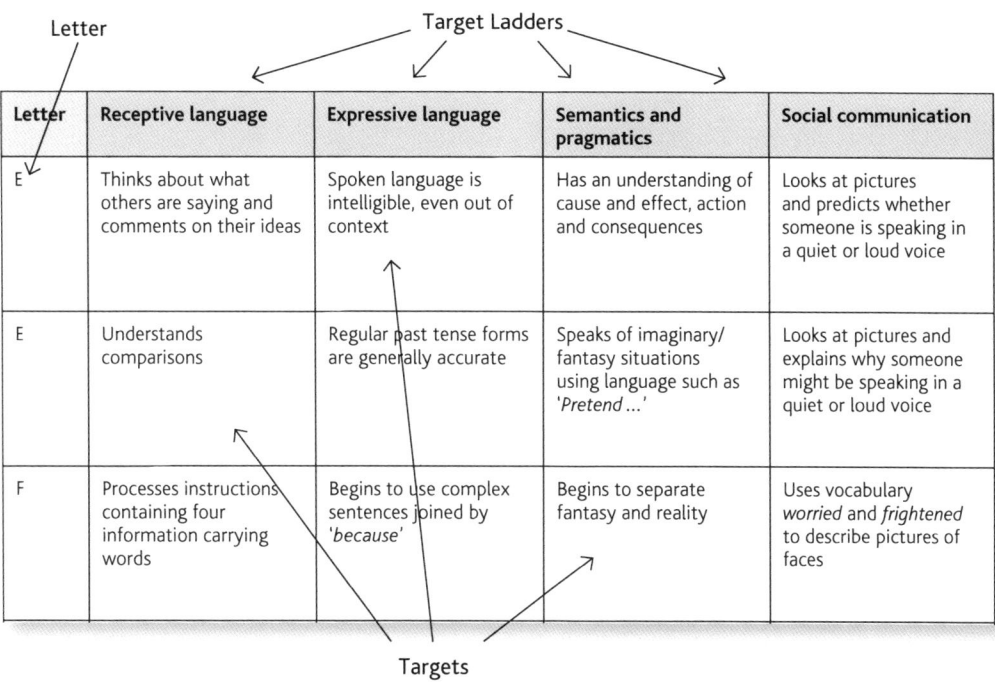

Fig. 5: Part of the Target Ladders table for **Aspect 3: Auditory processing for communication** showing how targets are structured in the ladders.

Although within each Target Ladder rows with the same letter are similar, this is not the case between the different Target Ladders. So a child may have an A target in one ladder and a G target in another. Some of the Target Ladders start at a very early developmental level, whereas others assume a level of competence even in the A rows. Again, use your professional judgement and be guided by the child's abilities and needs. The letters are simply there to help you to identify targets which are at approximately the same developmental level within the same Target Ladder.

The targets are all written in positive language. This is to support you when you look through them to find out what the child *can already* do. Use them as the basis of the target you set for the child.

As you track the statements through each ladder, identifying what the child can already do, be aware of missed steps. If a child has missed one of the steps, further progress up that ladder may be insecure. Many children learn to mask the missed step, using developing skills in other areas to help them, but the time may come when the missed step will cause difficulties.

Activities and strategies to achieve the targets

In the Target Ladders on pages 42–83, targets are listed on left-hand pages. The corresponding right-hand pages offer ideas for activities or strategies that you might use to help to achieve the targets. These are suggestions only – but many have been used successfully in classrooms and are accepted good practice. The activities or strategies are shown at the point in the developmental process at which they are likely to make the most impact.

The suggested activities can often be adapted to work for a range of targets within this stage of the ladder. For this reason, activities are generally not linked to individual targets.

How to set targets: a four-step summary

1. **Use Fig. 4 on page 34 to identify the one or two Aspects of working memory or auditory processing that are most challenging for the child.** Please use the list of indicators on pages 21–23 for guidance.

2. **Use the Target Ladders tables on pages 42–83**, to pinpoint specific targets for the child to work towards. Look at easier targets in the same ladder to ensure that the child has achieved all of those.

3. **Photocopy the relevant targets page** so that you can:
   - highlight and date those the child can already do;
   - identify the next priorities.

4. **Use the Record of Progress sheet on page 39 to create a copy of the targets for the child or their parents.**

Making the most of Target Ladders

You may find the following tips helpful when setting your targets.

- Talk to the child about what they would like to improve; a target that the child wants to improve is more likely to be successful.
- Discuss targets with the child's parents/carers.
- Think about your main concerns about that child's learning.
- Once you have identified the Aspect, identify the most beneficial Target Ladder.
  - Look for any 'missed steps', and target those first. The child is likely to find success fairly quickly and will be motivated to continue to try to reach new targets.
  - Talk to the child and agree an appropriate target based on your skills inventory. Again, targets which the child is aware of tend to be achieved most quickly and are motivational.
- The target does not have to be the lowest unachieved statement in any ladder: use your professional judgement and knowledge of the child to identify the most useful and important target for the child.
- No child will follow all of the targets in precisely the order listed. Use your

professional judgement, and your knowledge about what the child can already do, to identify the most appropriate target and be realistic in your expectations. There may be some zigzagging up and down a Target ladder.
- When setting targets, always ask yourself practical questions:
  - What can I put in place in order to enable the child to meet the targets?
  - Which people and resources are available to support the child?
  - What is the likelihood of a child achieving a target within the next half-term?
  - Which targets have been agreed with other children in the class?

It is important that the targets you set are realistic considering the time, the adult support and the resources available.

Once you have identified what the child can already achieve, continue to highlight and update the sheets each time the child achieves a new target. Celebrate progress with the child while, at the same time, constantly checking to ensure that previously achieved targets remain secure. If any target becomes insecure, revisit it briefly, without setting a formal target, in order to give the child an opportunity to consolidate the skill without feeling that they are going backwards in their achievements.

Records of Progress

Creating a Record of Progress

If the child can communicate confidently, arrange to meet with them and their parents and ask them first to tell you what they are good at. When working with the child, you may need to adapt the immediate visual environment to support the child. For example, any task sheet may need to be simplified and/or enlarged. You may wish to colour-code the chart or consider carefully the colour of paper and text, or the style of font. Record their responses on the Record of Progress (RoP). A blank form is supplied for you to copy on page 39. Ask the child and their parents then to tell you which areas they would most like to improve.

If your school operates a Pupil Passport system, then you may want to amend the RoP form, but you will nonetheless need a sheet that can be annotated and amended.

As you add one or two more targets, talk to the child and their parents to check that they agree that each target is relevant and that they understand what they will need to do to achieve their targets. Targets that children do not know or care about are much harder for them to achieve. Limit the number of targets to a maximum of three. Remember, you do not need to use the precise wording of the targets given in this book: adapt the words to match the maturity and understanding of the learner. Monitor the impact of any intervention (see page 41) and review at regular intervals – at least half-termly – to see if there is an impact. If not, consider whether a different intervention would be more effective.

Principles for the effective use of an RoP include the following:

- The form must be 'live'. The child will need to have access to it at all times, as will all adults who work with the child, in order that it can be referred to, amended and updated regularly. Ensure that the child's parents/carers have a copy. If you think that the child is likely to lose or destroy their RoP, make a photocopy so that you can supply another.
- Together with the child, you have identified their priority areas to focus on. Management and support for these should be consistent across the school day and from all adults.
- As soon as each target has been achieved, according to the success criteria you agreed, the form should be dated and a 'next step' considered.
- When you set up the RoP, agree a review date which is ideally about half a term ahead and no more than one term ahead. Do not wait until this date to identify that targets have been achieved, but on this date review progress towards all targets – or identified next steps – and agree new targets.
- If a target has not been achieved, consider why not. If possible, try a different approach to meeting the target. Having the same target over and over is likely to bore the child and put them off following their RoP.

RECORD OF PROGRESS

Name _____ Class _____ Date agreed _____ RoP number: _____ Review date _____

I am good at	My targets are	I will know that I have achieved my target when I can	Date when I achieved my target	Next steps
I would like to be better at				
It helps me when				

Targets approved by: Pupil _____ Teacher _____

SENCO _____ Parent/Carer _____

Monitoring a Record of Progress

In order to ensure that your Record of Progress (RoP) is used effectively, you need to monitor progress towards the targets each time you offer support. Use a monitoring sheet; a photocopiable example is given on page 41.

- Use a separate sheet – copied on to a different colour of paper – for each target.
- Write the child's name at the top of the sheet and the target underneath.
- On each occasion when someone works with the child towards the target, they should write the smaller, more specific target that you are working towards *during this session* in the Target box.
- They should then write a comment. On each occasion the child achieves the target during the session and then back in class, tick the box.

The intention is that these sheets should be used to create a cumulative record of a child's progress towards their target. The evidence here can be used to assess the impact of an intervention in order that its appropriateness can be evaluated swiftly and any additional actions can be taken promptly.

What precisely you record will depend on the type of support being offered and the nature of the target.

- If you are delivering a planned intervention, make a record of the unit/page/activity and a comment about the learning the child demonstrated. For example, a comment relating to a target about the child's ability to remember a string of items may be: *'Told me the three correct items but did not recall the colours in serial order'*.
- If you are offering support in the classroom, you might want to comment on the child's learning over a few lessons. Focus on what the child has achieved in the lessons and whether the learning is secure.
- As a general principle, aim to include more positive than negative comments, and always try to balance a negative with a positive comment.

At the half-termly review of the RoP, collect together all of the monitoring sheets and look at the frequency of the comments against each target as well as the learning they reflect. If a child has had absences, or an intervention has not happened as often as planned, consider what impact that has had on the effectiveness of the intervention. If the intervention has gone as planned, look at the progress charted and ask yourself these questions:

- Is it swift enough? Is the intervention helping this child to close the gap? Is the adult working with the child the best person for the job?
- Is this the best intervention? Is there anything else you can reasonably do in school?
- What should happen next? If the intervention was successful, do you continue it, develop it, consolidate it or change to a different target?

At the end of the process, create a new RoP with the child and their parents/carers and use a new monitoring sheet.

Records of Progress

Monitoring the progress of _____ towards meeting the

target of _____

Date	Today's Target	Comment	Achieved			

The Target Ladders

Aspect 1: Auditory processing and exploring sound

Letter	Pitch and volume	Beat, rhythm, location	Making sounds	Background noise
A	Spontaneously shouts and whispers during play activities	Watches and tracks with eyes as someone moves back and forth across a room playing a musical instrument	Plays with position of tongue on request (e.g. sticks it out, licks, wiggles)	Registers and turns towards a familiar person's voice in a quiet environment
A	Imitates an adult whispering and talking in a loud voice	Joins in clapping a regular beat	Plays with position of lips (e.g. kisses own hand, sucks through a straw, blows bubbles, moves from smile to pursed lips and back)	Responds to simple requests in a quiet situation
B	Tolerates loud noise in the playground with warning and support/ears covered	Eyes shut: head follows a musical instrument as the player moves back and forth across a room	Plays with position of jaw (e.g. opens and closes mouth, moves bottom jaw to left and right)	Turns towards the speaker when own name is called in a quiet environment
B	Tolerates loud noise in the classroom without support/ears covered	Joins in with clapping a simple, repeated rhythm	Uses voice to gain attention	Picks up a named object/ points to a named picture in a quiet situation
C	Tolerates assemblies with warning and support/ears covered	Eyes shut: musical instrument plays in a corner of the room; child swivels and points to the location	Identifies how tongue, lips, jaw and teeth are used in exploring and chewing food	Responds to simple requests in a quiet situation when the speaker is speaking quietly
C	Tolerates assemblies without support/ears covered	Imitates clapping a simple repeated rhythm	Uses voice to gain a specific person's attention	Turns towards the speaker when own name is called in a noisy environment
D	Understands the difference between making a loud sound and a quiet one	Eyes shut: can say whether a tambourine or triangle is heard and point to the location	Uses slow and quick breaths to blow paint across a piece of paper with a straw	Responds to simple requests in a quiet situation but with some background noise
D	Uses a visual to point to loudness and quietness of class environment	Eyes shut: can say whether a tambourine, triangle or jingle bells is heard and point to the location	Drinks water from a bottle with a sports cap	Responds to simple requests in a noisy environment

Suggested activities or strategies

Using visual scales

Children with APD generally work better with visuals than with language. Let them play with a voice recording app which shows the volume of the voice. Ask them to listen carefully to relate the sound they hear/feel to the volume control. Make a copy of the volume control of the type you have used and show where on the control each voice-type is shown. Teach the child to modulate their voice according to how it feels and to use the visual to show how loud they think their voice is and how loud your voice is.

Give instructions to the child in quiet places but increasingly make your voice quieter.

Harbour and lighthouses

Play with a group of children in a large empty space. One child (the ship) is blindfolded (or pulls a woollen hat down over their eyes). Another (the safe harbour) stands at the edge of the space and plays a triangle. Others (rocks with lighthouses on them) sit on the floor. The ship has to reach the harbour. If they are in danger of crashing into a rock the lighthouse on the rock emits a warning sound so the ship can steer safely through the rocks.

As children become more proficient at playing the game, add in other distractor instruments (e.g. tambourine, jingle bells) as enemy harbours: the ship still has to get to the safe harbour of the triangle.

Helping tactile/oral defensiveness

If there is a serious problem, you are advised to seek support from a specialist speech and language therapist or occupational therapist who will give advice about a suitable programme of work. If, however, there is some defensiveness, but it is not interfering with the child's nutrition, you can support them in school. You might want to ask the parents to take the child to a dentist first, to ensure that sensitivities are not due to the health of teeth and gums.

First, consider whether the child has a general tactile defensiveness to textures such as sand, glue, finger paint or, if orally defensive, whether the problem is due to low oral tone leading to poor awareness of what is happening in the mouth.

- Check the child can label all the parts of their mouth: lips, tongue, cheek, gums, teeth.
- Model giving yourself a gum and inner-cheek massage, feeling all around the mouth, asking the child to listen to the different sounds your finger makes on your gums and teeth. Sing any note while you massage your inner cheek and listen to how the sound changes as you move your cheek. Ask the child to give themselves a gum massage like the one you did.
- The child may benefit from using different shapes and textures of chew tools or 'chewelry' which will help to develop oral tone.
- Let the child play with dental tongue depressors. Ask them to explore how it feels to press different places on the tongue. Get them to try saying words and singing notes while depressing their tongue at different places. How does pressing the tongue affect the sounds and words?
- Make faces at each other in a mirror: one person makes a face for the other to copy.
- Blow bubbles, whistles, swannee whistles, mouth organs.
- Suck and blow water through different types and lengths of straws.
- Mix paint with water and washing-up liquid. Blow bubbles and press paper gently on top to make bubble prints.
- Make trails of paint by blowing it across a piece of paper with a straw. Try using different types of straw and different kinds of breaths: slow and deep or quick and shallow.
- Drink from different kinds of cup and bottle, including sports bottles.

Emphasise that the child should only put food in their mouth unless they are given special permission to put anything else inside their mouth.

Aspect 1: Visual memory skills

Letter	Pitch and volume	Beat, rhythm, location	Making sounds	Background noise
E	Uses a visual to point to loudness and quietness of an adult voice	Joins in tapping the rhythm of a familiar character's name	Joins in with making different voice sounds (e.g. humming, clicking, puffing, squeaky)	Demonstrates being a good listener in a quiet room
E	Uses a visual to point to loudness and quietness of own voice	Uses tokens to represent the number of words in a short phrase (up to three words)	Imitates animal noises	Explains how ears, eyes and hands all contribute to being a good listener
F	Responds to a visual to make voice louder or quieter	Identifies a familiar character's name from a tapped rhythm (from two pictures shown)	Imitates making different voice sounds (e.g. humming, clicking, puffing, squeaky)	Responds to simple requests when working in a small group
F	Responds to requests to speak in a louder or quieter voice	Uses tokens to represent the number of words in a short sentence (up to five words)	Makes animals noises when shown a picture of an animal	Demonstrates being a good listener in a quiet area near a noisier area
G	With an adult, looks at people in school and identifies whether they are using a loud or a quiet voice	Identifies a familiar character's name from a tapped rhythm (from three pictures shown)	On a sound walk, identifies people using the right amount of volume for the context	Follows adult directions while participating in an activity in a small group
G	Starts to develop vocabulary to talk about reasons for using a loud or quiet voice	Identifies a familiar animal name from a tapped rhythm (from three pictures shown)	On a sound walk, follows instructions to identify and copy sounds which are loud or soft	Responds to other children while participating in an activity in a small group
H	Imitates an adult's pitch of voice (e.g. talking in a high squeaky or deep low voice)	Imitates clapping syllables in one-syllable words or two-syllable compound words (e.g. *hair, hairbrush*)	On a sound walk, follows instructions to identify and copy sounds which are long or short	Joins in conversations with a small group in a quiet area near a noisier area
H	Uses hand to indicate the pitch of a voice (e.g. hand held low for deep low voice and hand held high for a high squeaky voice)	Imitates clapping syllables of two-syllable animal names	On a sound walk, follows instructions to identify and copy sounds which are high or low	Participates in show and tell in a small group in a quiet area near a noisier area

Suggested activities or strategies

Count up

Children need to be able to separate running speech into individual words before they will be able to identify syllables of phonemes.

Give the child some counters and a piece of landscape A5 paper. Ask the child to listen carefully while you say some words and then to put counters on the paper to show how many words you said.

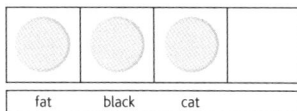

Start with simple noun phrases using one-syllable words only (e.g. '*black cat*', '*red ball*', '*good book*', '*cup of tea*'). Over several sessions, build up to longer sentences which include more than one syllable (e.g. '*Do you like buttercups?*'; '*That computer is very old*'; '*Our science lesson was interesting*').

Long and short

If you or the child have a mobile phone, listen to a range of ring tones (many internet sites offer this too). Talk about whether the sounds are long sounds, or short ones. Listen to sound clips of environmental sounds online (e.g. at the British Library's sound collection www.sounds.bl.uk). Identify sounds which are long (e.g. sirens, engines, waterfalls) and short (e.g. squeaking, hammering, dropping things).

Go for a sound walk around the school listening for duration of different sounds.

Get that rhythm

Depending on the age of the child, make a list of characters' names from songs, films or books. Help the child to find an illustration of each of the characters (e.g. Harry Potter, Ron, Dumbledore, Hagrid, Hermione, Snape, etc.). As you say each of the names, gently clap/tap/beat a drum to show the syllabic structure of the names. Show the children two characters. If you clap one of their names can the child tell you which one? Can they clap a name for you to?

Show them images linked to compound words (e.g. lighthouse, butterfly, homework, photograph, goalkeeper, handwriting, headteacher, watermelon). If you clap a rhythm, can the child clap the rhythm again and show you a picture that has that rhythm?

Show and tell

Ask a small group of children to bring a special thing into school they would like to tell you about. Work with the group in a quiet room with the door open. Remind children of the rules of good listening: *eyes* looking, *ears* listening, *hands* and *feet* still, *brain* working. (Use reminder visuals if you can.) Ask each child in turn to talk about their special thing while all the rest of the children listen and think of a question to ask at the end.

As children become more confident at speaking and listening show them the words: *what, why, when, how, who, where*. Ask the speaker to include information about what their chosen thing is; why they chose it; and information about one of the other *wh-* words (e.g. *who* gave it to them; *where* they keep it; *how* they use it). Ask the listeners to listen out for information about three *wh-* words and to think of questions beginning with one of the other *wh-* words.

Doh, re, mi

Let children play with glockenspiels as well as different-sized cymbals so they learn to see low and high notes as well as hear them. Show children how they can grow upwards from low notes, where they are crouching down, to the highest notes, where they are standing on tiptoe. (If children prefer not to move their whole bodies, show them how to hold their hands from low to high.) Model talking in a deep growly voice while you are crouched and a high-pitched squeaky voice while you are standing on tiptoe. Can the child imitate you? Older children might like to learn some of the doh, re, mi hand positions (e.g. www.sing4me.ca/curwen.htm).

Ask the child to shut their eyes, listen to you talking in a low voice, an ordinary voice and a high voice. Can they show you where your voice is? Let them make the voices while your eyes are shut so that you can show where their voice is.

Aspect 1: Visual memory skills

Letter	Pitch and volume	Beat, rhythm, location	Making sounds	Background noise
I	Looks at pictures and predicts whether someone is speaking in a quiet or loud voice	Imitates clapping syllables in two- or three-syllable compound words (e.g. *hairbrush, buttercup*)	Repeats a string of nonsense syllables starting with a long consonant sound (e.g. *ma, ma, ma, ma; so, so, so, so*)	Follows adult directions to a small group in a quiet classroom
I	Copies different tones of voice to express different emotions	Imitates clapping syllables in three-syllable animal names (e.g. *crocodile, chimpanzee*)	Repeats a string of nonsense syllables starting with a short consonant sound (e.g. *ba, ba, ba, ba; ti, ti, ti, ti*)	Participates in conversation in a quiet classroom
J	Looks at pictures and explains why someone might be speaking in a high or low voice	Listens to syllabic pattern (up to three syllables) and identifies all animals from a choice given with that syllabic pattern	Joins in reciting alliterative phrases or sentences	Follows adult directions in normal classroom noise
J	Changes tone of voice to express emotions	Listens to a rhythmic pattern and identifies the opening line of a familiar song or rhyme	Claps when hears a repeated sound in alliterative phrases or sentences	Participates in conversation in normal classroom noise
K	With support, in role-play, uses volume of voice appropriately	Independently claps syllables in one- or two-syllable animal names	Identifies the key sound in alliterative phrases or sentences	Listens during whole-class teaching sessions
K	With support, in role-play, uses pitch of voice appropriately	Uses counters to represent syllables (up to three)	Identifies an animal from a choice of three that could be described with an alliterative adjective (e.g. *happy hungry hippo*)	Listens and joins in group work in a busy classroom
L	Uses and responds to pitch of voice appropriately	Independently claps syllables in two- or three-syllable animal names	Repeats a string of rhyming syllables (e.g. *man, fan, pan, lan*)	Hears and follows instructions from teachers, even when there is background noise
L	Varies volume of voice according to context	Uses counters to represent up to five syllables (e.g. *hip-po-pot-a-mus*)	Repeats a string of alliterative syllables (e.g. *ban, bin, bon, bun, ben*)	Filters background noise effectively

Suggested activities or strategies

Which voice?
Take some digital photographs of the child talking at different times of the school day, including in the dining hall and outside. (If you can't take photos of the individual child, take photos of their classmates when you know that the child was around.) Talk about the pitch and volume that were used in each of the photographs. Ask the child to describe the pitch and volume they used and talk about whether or not they were appropriate.

Animal names
Play games using pictures of animals with different numbers of syllables from one (e.g. *dog*, *cat*, *swan*) to two (e.g. *warthog*, *zebra*), to three (e.g. *antelope*, *elephant*, *crocodile*), to four (e.g. *rhinoceros*, *alligator*, *armadillo*), to five (e.g. *hippopotamus*, *tyrannosaurus*, *komodo dragon*). Once the child can identify the animals, play games like:

- **syllable count**: show two or three pictures with different number of syllables (e.g. *sheep*, *tiger*, *elephant*). Use taps, beats or counters to show the number of syllables for the animal you're thinking of. Can your partner work out the animal?
- **syllable sort**: time the child as they sort the animal pictures into sets with the same number of syllables;
- **syllable Snap**: say '*Snap*' when you see two animals with the same number of syllables;
- **syllabic memory**: find pairs of pictures with the same number of syllables.

Whose voice?
Take photos and make an audio recording of times during the school day when the child should be listening (e.g. in assembly, class listening time, group work time, paired work time, independent working). Show the child the photos. For each one, can they tell you whose voice is the most important at that time? Play the audio recordings. Can the child put their hand up when the most important voice is speaking? Can they tell you what that person is saying?

Take a message
If you can, speak on the phone to the child when the child is in the school office, surrounded by normal office sounds. Give the child two messages. For the first, make sure that your mouth is close to the microphone of your phone. For the second, move the phone around a bit so your voice will be less clear.

When you can talk normally to the child, see how much of each of the messages they managed to understand. Can they tell you which message was harder? Can they explain why? Talk about what they did and didn't get right. Discuss strategies for 'closing the gaps' in words that are not completely heard, such as:

- thinking about what the message *might* be about and listening hard to see if you can hear words which are about the topic;
- listening for the nouns and verbs and not worrying too much initially about other words;
- listening for the words the speaker emphasises and says more clearly – those are likely to be important words;
- listening primarily to the first syllable.

Tongue-twisters
Tongue-twisters and alliterative sentences are an easy and enjoyable way to help to tune in the ears to hearing sounds in words and are comparatively easy to adapt for individual children's ages and interests. From traditional tongue-twisters (e.g. *round and round the ragged rock the ragged rascal ran*) to simple alliterative sentences (e.g. *Shawn the sheep was shaving*) and phrases (e.g. *ten tiny toes*) the challenge is:

- to identify the repeated sound;
- to count repetitions of the main sound;
- to hear the target sound at the beginning, middle and end of words (e.g. *grimy diggers dug up my garden*);
- to suggest other words you could include in the tongue-twisters;
- to create new alliterative phrases and tongue-twisters.

Aspect 1: Auditory processing and exploring sound

Aspect 2: Auditory processing for phonological development

Letter	Identifying sounds	Speech sounds	Blending sounds	Rhyme
A	Listens to a pre-recorded environmental sound and selects a picture from a choice of three very different sounds (e.g. bee, tractor, rainfall)	Listens to isolated speech sounds with movement and/or picture prompts (e.g. /b/, /m/)	Identifies what is at the front or beginning of a queue of objects	Listens to nursery rhymes/rhymes and requests favourites
A	Listens to a pre-recorded environmental sound and selects a picture from a choice of three more similar sounds (e.g. tractor, motorbike, domestic car)	Imitates isolated speech sounds using movement and/or a picture prompt	Identifies what is at the back or end of a queue of objects	Joins in with some familiar nursery rhymes/rhymes
B	Listens to two pre-recorded environmental sounds and sequences pictures to show the order they were heard in	Makes isolated speech sounds using movement and/or picture prompts	Repeats the word at the beginning of a 3–4 word phrase or sentence (e.g. *Good morning, Charlie.*)	Joins in with saying rhyming words at the end of familiar rhyming couplets
B	Listens to three pre-recorded environmental sounds and sequences pictures to show the order they were heard in	Identifies isolated speech sounds using movement and/or a picture prompt	Repeats the word at the end of a 3–4 word phrase or sentence (e.g. *Black cats like sleeping.*)	Says rhyming words at the end of familiar rhyming couplets
C	Says whether two VC* nonsense syllables are the same (e.g. *oop*, *oop*) or different (e.g. *arg*, *arb*)	Says whether two speech sounds are the same (e.g. /k , k/) or different (e.g. /k, m/)	Identifies the 'odd one out' when shown two pictures beginning with the same sound and a phonologically dissimilar distractor (e.g. *cup*, *man*, *cake*)	Joins in with generating strings of rhyming words (including nonsense words) (e.g. *pen*, *when*, *sen*, *len*, *hen*)
C	Imitates pairs of VC nonsense syllables which are sometimes the same (e.g. *owp*, *owp*) and sometimes different (e.g. *owp*, *owk*)	Imitates pairs of speech sounds which are sometimes the same (e.g. *ai*, *ay*) and sometimes different (e.g. *ai*, *ow*)	Identifies the 'odd one out' when shown two pictures beginning with the same sound and a phonologically similar distractor (e.g. *ten*, *dog*, *tape*)	Independently generates strings of rhyming words (including nonsense words)
D	Says whether two VC real words are the same (e.g. *in*, *in*) or different (e.g. *in*, *on*; *in*, *it*)	Imitates short vowel sounds in isolation (e.g. vowels in: p*a*t, p*e*t, p*i*t, p*o*t, p*u*t, p*u*tt, P*e*ter)	Points to an object beginning with a given sound	Listens and joins in when variations of familiar rhymes are said with new rhyming words
D	Imitates pairs of VC real words which are sometimes the same (e.g. *at*, *at*) and sometimes different (e.g. *at*, *app*)	Imitates long vowel sounds in isolation (e.g. vowels in b*ai*t, b*ea*t, b*i*te, b*oa*t, b*oo*t, B*a*rt, B*e*rt, b*ough*t, br*ow*, b*oy*, b*ear*, b*ee*r)	Says the sound at the beginning of a word	Suggests new rhyming words for variations of familiar rhymes

*C = consonant   V = vowel

Suggested activities or strategies

Say it with mirrors

Use mirrors while you model and imitate sounds. If a child's ability to know which sounds they are listening for and reproducing is impaired in any way, visual support is invaluable – as well as great fun.

Play with making and copying silly faces in the mirrors, then add sound effects. Initially, they don't need to be recognisable sounds, just a silly noise to accompany a funny face.

When you move onto making speech sounds, continue to use mirrors. Encourage the child to rub their gums and tongues before you begin as this helps to sensitize the child to where in the mouth they are making the sounds.

Same or different?

Check that the idea of same or different is secure using pictures. Show:

- two pictures of the same object;
- two pictures of objects that are similar but not the same (e.g. a blue brush and a red brush; a small red ball and a bigger red ball);
- two different views of an object: the pictures are different, but the object is the same.

Once you can be sure that the child knows and understands the meaning of same and different, move on to explore sounds. Use the chart below to ensure that when you play 'same or different?' with consonant and vowel sounds:

- initially choose two sounds that are different in both where and how they are made: consonants which are very different (e.g. /s, g/) or two vowels that are very different (e.g. /i, ar/);
- then, as the child gets better at the game you can choose sounds that are more similar so they either differ in where they are made (e.g. /p, k/ or /i, a/) or how they are made (e.g. /k, g/ or /a, o/).

I spy

As children become familiar with hearing the sound at the beginning of a word, play games like I Spy.

- Initially only give a choice of three pictures (use the chart below to ensure that the sounds are very different) (e.g. *I spy with my little eye something beginning with /p/* when the choices are a dog, a nut and a pan).
- Then give choices that are phonologically more similar (e.g. *I spy with my little eye something beginning with /p/* when the choices are a bat, a tin and a pin).
- Then widen the possibilities of words to a simple picture.

Rhyming variations

This activity is easiest to do with nursery rhymes, but you could use any silly poem with rhyming couplets. Say the first line of the couplet, with a different final word, then a variation on the second line of the couplet to lead the child to the best choice of rhyming words. Offer three pictures to select from (e.g. *Humpty Dumpty sat on a box/hat/chair, Humpty Dumpty saw a (bear/fox/cat)*).

Aspect 2: Auditory processing for phonological development

	Lips	Tongue at front of mouth	Tongue at back of mouth		Tongue at front of mouth	Tongue at back of mouth	
Voiceless*	p f	t s	k	Tongue high (close)	pit peat	put boot	
Voiced*	b v	d z	g	Tongue mid	pet	port	
Nasal	m	n	ng	Tongue low (open)	pat	pot part	
Liquid	r		l				

* Voiced or voiceless refers to whether there are vibrations in the larynx (throat). Voiced sounds like /z/ have vibrations, whereas voiceless sounds like /s/ don't. All vowels, liquids and nasals are voiced.

Aspect 2: Auditory processing for phonological development

Letter	Identifying sounds	Speech sounds	Blending sounds	Rhyme
E	Says whether two CV* nonsense words are the same (e.g. *foo, foo; foo*) or different (e.g. *noo*)	Uses an appropriate short vowel sound when saying single-syllable words	Listens to an adult saying sounds in a CVC (consonant-vowel-consonant) word (e.g. *h-a-t*) and selects the appropriate object from a choice of three	Makes pairs of rhyming words from a set of six cards (representing three pairs)
E	Imitates pairs of CV nonsense words which are sometimes the same (e.g. *pow, pow*) and sometimes different (e.g. *pow, dow*)	Uses an appropriate long vowel sound when saying single-syllable words	Imitates an adult saying sounds in a CVC word (e.g. *m-o-p*) and selects the appropriate object from a choice of three	Makes pairs of rhyming words from a set of ten cards (representing five pairs)
F	Says whether two CV real words are the same (e.g. *pay, pay*) or different (e.g. *pay, Kay*)	Imitates an appropriate initial sound when saying single-syllable words	In response to a word spoken by an adult, uses 'phonic fingers'** to represent sounds in a CVC word (e.g. *f-i-sh*)	With support, completes a range of simple rhyming activities
F	Imitates pairs of CV words which are sometimes the same (e.g. *key, key*) and sometimes different (e.g. *key, tea*)	Uses an appropriate initial sound when saying single-syllable words	In response to a picture, uses 'phonic fingers' to represent sounds in a CVC word (e.g. *sh-ee-p*)	Independently completes a range of simple rhyming activities
G	Says whether two CVC nonsense syllables are the same (e.g. *dorp, dorp*) or different (e.g. *dorp, dort; dorp, corp*)	Imitates an appropriate final sound when saying single-syllable words	Identifies two objects that end with the same sound out of a set of three	Plays games such as rhyming Lotto and rhyming Snap with adult support
G	Imitates pairs of CVC nonsense syllables which are sometimes the same (e.g. *pard, pard*) and sometimes different (e.g. *pard, tard; pard, parg*)	Uses an appropriate final sound when saying single-syllable words	Identifies the 'odd one out' when shown two pictures ending with the same sound and a phonologically similar distractor	Plays games such as rhyming Lotto and rhyming Snap with a group of other children
H	Says whether two CVC real words are the same (e.g. *seat, seat*) or different (e.g. *seat, seek; seat, peat*)	Imitates CVC words accurately	Points to an object which ends with a given sound	Can say whether two words rhyme, including semantic distractors (e.g. *cat, mouse; cat, mat*)
H	Imitates pairs of CVC words which are sometimes the same (e.g. *wheat, wheat*) and sometimes different (e.g. *wheat, week; wheat, seat; wheat, white*)	Pronounces all sounds accurately when saying CVC words	Points to an object with a given vowel sound	Can say whether two words rhyme, including phonological distractors (e.g. *cat, map; cat, hat*)

*C = consonant   V = vowel

**'phonic fingers' = where you hold up one finger to represent each sound

Suggested activities or strategies

Imitating speech sounds and syllables

When you introduce mimicking speech sounds use the progression of imitating:

- the sound in isolation (e.g. /f/);
- a nonsense syllable *ending* with the sound (e.g. *oof, eef, owf, urf*);
- the target sound at the *end* of a short real word (e.g. *if, off, niff, laugh*);
- the target sound at the *beginning* of a nonsense syllable (e.g. *fee, foo, foi, fow*);
- the target sound at the *beginning* of a short real word (e.g. *fit, fan, fun*);
- the target sound between two vowels in the middle of a nonsense word (e.g. *eefee, arfar, aifoo*);
- the target sound between two vowels in the middle of a real word (e.g. *orphan, soften, sofa, toffee*).

Nonsense words and syllables are always introduced before 'real' words and syllables because the child has no muscle-memory of saying a nonsense word, and there is no meaning attached to it, so the child is less likely to make habitual sound production errors.

Ensure that the child is secure and accurate at one stage before moving onto the next.

See the Sound – Visual Phonics programme (www.seethesound.org)

See the Sound – Visual Phonics was created for children with hearing impairments. It works well for children who have APD because they don't always process sounds in the same way as their peers do so the mainstream phonics lesson may be mystifying to them. Visual Phonics is a system of hand shapes and written symbols to represent the sounds in English. The hand shapes are often linked to the signing alphabet and some bear some relationship to the written letter shape. Many of the signs are helpfully made to remind the child where in the mouth the sound is made (e.g. /k/ is represented by thumb and fingers forming a 'c' shape by the throat, to show that the sound is made at the back of the mouth). You can find videos and posters online, many of which are posted by speech therapists.

Beginning to blend

When you begin to teach blending, whisper the sounds, elongating them as much as you can. At this stage, children don't have to read the words, just to hear them, so a word like *mouse* or *moon* is no harder than *cat* but has more sounds that can be drawn out.

When you choose pictures for the blending activities, use the chart on page 49 to ensure that the words do not have similar sounds (e.g. blend /f -i -sh/ and show pictures of a cart, a train and a fish). As the child gets better at hearing and blending the sounds, make the pictures more similar so you might offer a fish, a ship and a fin.

Repeating words

For these activities, CVC words can have long or short vowels – they are spoken, not read.

Before the child tries to say CVC words, ask them to imitate each of the words as you name the pictures for a game. Do not use pictures for the game that the child does not immediately say accurately. You will need to rehearse those words separately using ideas from page 49. Let the child say all the words during the game, but if any are said with errors, ask the child to imitate you saying the word before you place those pictures in a pile to revisit.

- **Magnetic fishing.** Attach a metal paper clip to each picture and let the child fish for them with a small magnet on a string tied to a paintbrush. Let the child say all the words, but if any are said with errors, ask the child to imitate you saying the word. Place those pictures in a pile to revisit.
- **Feel it first.** Use objects instead of pictures. Before you play the game, ask the child to say the word for each object and let them explore the object with their fingers. Put all the objects in a box, a bag or behind a screen and ask the child to identify them only by touch.

Aspect 2: Auditory processing for phonological development

Letter	Identifying sounds	Speech sounds	Blending sounds	Rhyme
I	Imitates an adult saying the sounds in a CCVC* or CVCC word (e.g. *d-e-s-k* or *c-l-ow-n*) and selects the appropriate object from a choice of three	Imitates CCVC words (e.g. *flag*, *snail*), saying all the sounds clearly	Says if two words are the same when one may be missing the initial sound (e.g. *cake*, *ache*; *ball*, *all*)	When the words are spoken aloud, identifies the non-rhyming 'odd one out' from a set of three pictures where the words are spoken and the distractor is semantic (e.g. *sock*, *shoe*, *clock*)
I	In response to a word spoken by an adult, uses 'phonic fingers'** to represent sounds in a CCVC or CVCC word (e.g. *s-w-i-m*, *ch-i-m-p*)	Imitates CVCC words (e.g. *tent*, *lamp*), saying all the sounds clearly	Says if two words are the same when one may be missing the final sound (e.g. *sort*, *sore*; *page*, *pay*)	Without hearing the words, identifies the non-rhyming 'odd one out' from a set of three pictures where the distractor is semantic (e.g. *sock*, *shoe*, *clock*)
J	Imitates an adult saying sounds in a CCVCC (e.g. *d-r-i-n-k*) or CCCVC word (e.g. *s-t-r-ee-t*) and selects the appropriate object from a choice of three	Imitates CCVCC words (e.g. *stamp*, *blend*), saying all the sounds clearly	Says if two words are the same when one may be missing one of adjacent initial consonants (e.g. *drain*, *rain*; *plate*, *late*)	When the words are spoken aloud, identifies the non-rhyming 'odd one out' from a set of three pictures where the words are spoken and the distractor is phonological (e.g. *cat*, *mat*, *map*)
J	In response to a word spoken by an adult, uses 'phonic fingers' to represent sounds in a CCVCC or CCCVC word (e.g. *g-r-ou-n-d*, *s-t-r-i-ng*)	Imitates CCCVC words (e.g. *stream*, *spring*) saying all the sounds clearly	Says if two words are the same when one may be missing one of adjacent final consonants (e.g. *tent*, *ten*; *fist*, *fit*)	Without hearing the words, identifies the non-rhyming 'odd one out' from a set of three pictures where the distractor is phonological (e.g. *cat*, *mat*, *map*)
K	Identifies similarities between pairs of heard CVC words (e.g. *cat*, *hat*; *cat*, *cap*; *cat*, *cot*)	Imitates two-syllable compound words, saying all the sounds clearly	Makes a clear distinction in own speech between all sounds in CVC words	Learns a simple rhyme or some simple rhyming couplets by heart
K	Identifies differences between pairs of heard CVC words (e.g. *pat*, *pack*; *pat*, *cat*; *pat*, *pet*)	Imitates common two- and three-syllable words, saying all the sounds clearly	Identifies a full range of speech sounds in words	Learns variations based on a simple rhyme or some simple rhyming couplets by heart
L	Identifies differences between CVC words and CVCC/CCVC words (e.g. *ten*, *tent*; *cap*, *clap*)	Consistently uses appropriate sounds when saying single-syllable words	Makes a clear distinction in own speech between all sounds in words with adjacent consonants	Suggests new variations based on a simple rhyme or some simple rhyming couplets
L	Explains how you change a word to make a new one (e.g. *tap* into *tape* or *trap*)	Consistently uses appropriate sounds when saying multi-syllable words	Uses a full range of sounds accurately in own speech	Composes simple rhyming couplets

*C = consonant   V = vowel
**'phonic fingers' = where you hold up one finger to represent each sound

Suggested activities or strategies

Minimal pairs

Minimal pairs are pairs of words that differ in one sound only. Minimal pairs are usually single-syllable words which differ in:

- initial consonant (e.g. *pin, bin; fish, dish; ring, king; sell, shell*);
- final consonant (e.g. *cat, cap; cap, cab; on, off*);
- initial vowel (e.g. *an, in; off, if; all, owl*);
- final vowel (e.g. *car, cow; knee, now; law, low*);
- middle vowel (e.g. *cap, kip; cat, cot; pan, pin; bit, bat; plan, plane; strip, stripe*);
- initial adjacent consonant (e.g. *pain, plane; side, slide; fog, frog; swim, slim; grab, crab*);
- final adjacent consonant (e.g. *gull, gulp; fine, find; deck, desk*);
- middle consonant (e.g. *power, powder; winner, winter*).

Use minimal pairs for the child to:

- repeat, demonstrating clear articulation;
- explain what makes the words same/different;
- identify whether a pair of words/nonsense words is the same or minimally different;
- understand spelling conventions for pairs like *tap, tape; pin, pine; lick, like; hop, hope; tub, tube*.

Saying all the sounds

When you teach words with adjacent consonants (represented as CC) speak as clearly as you can. Ask the child to:

- repeat the word. Record your voice and theirs and ask them to check whether you both said all of the sounds in the same way.
- repeat all of the sounds as you segment the word (e.g. *stamp, s-t-a-m-p*);
- blend the word once you say the sounds (e.g. *s-t-a-m-p, stamp*);
- use the visual support of 'phonic fingers' (where you hold up one finger to represent each sound).

Blending

If a child experiences difficulties in blending sounds orally, try whispering them – it's easier to extend sounds when you whisper.

- First, whisper and extend the sounds in a CV (consonant-vowel), VC or CVC word which has fricatives (*s, z, sh, f, v, th, h*), approximants (*l, r, w, y*) and nasals (*n, m, ng*) such as:
  - *z-oo, s-ew, sh-oe, t-wo, f-our*;
  - *s-u-n, m-oo-n, f-i-sh, v-a-se, v-a-n, r-i-ng, s-i-ng, s-ie-ve, wha-le, th-i-n, y-e-ll, y-e-s, n-i-ne, f-i-ve, s-i-x*.

  For each word, show three pictures. Ask the child to say the sounds, say the word and point to the picture.

- Gradually introduce some word ending plosives (*p, b, t, d, k, g*) to make words like *r-e-d, sh-o-p, n-e-t, s-a-ck, s-o-ck, f-oo-t, r-oa-d, l-e-g*.
- Then use words that begin with a plosive but end with a fricative, approximants or nasal, (e.g. *t-oo-th, t-e-n, p-i-n, k-i-ng*).
- Finally use words that begin and end with plosives (e.g. *b-e-d, b-a-ck, t-i-ck, t-oa-d, t-ar-t*).

Word power

Improving the children's understanding of how changing the sounds of words impacts on the spelling of the words (and vice versa) will support their reading and spelling as well as tune their ears and voices into ensuring that minimal pairs sound different.

- Teach recognition of short vowels (those in the words *pat, pet, pit, pot, putt, put*) and long vowels (all the other vowels). This is particularly important because it determines whether or not consonants are doubled before suffixes are added (e.g. *hopping* (short), *hoping* (long); *tapping* (short), *taping* (long); *pinning* (short) *pining* (long); *licking* (short *ck* is always used in place of *kk*), *liking* (long)).
- Teach children to hear stressed and unstressed syllables. Whether a syllable is stressed or not can affect pronunciation – stressed often impacts on how the vowel is pronounced (e.g. the first syllable of *apron* is stressed whereas the first syllable of *about* is unstressed).
- As children develop language to talk about words and sounds, you can be more explicit as you discuss words, their pronunciation and their spelling.

Aspect 2: Auditory processing for phonological development

Aspect 3: Auditory processing for communication

Letter	Receptive language	Expressive language	Semantics and pragmatics	Social communication
A	Responds to commands at three-word level	Speaks in 3-4 word sentences	Asks simple questions to gain information	Engages in some shared/turn-taking activities
A	Understands 4+ word sentences	Uses noun plurals and uses -*ing* on verbs	Asks for permission to do things	Shares toys and resources with others
B	Responds to questions to identify objects (e.g. '*Which one do we sit on?*')	Asks simple questions (e.g. '*What are you doing?*')	Expresses own feelings through body language and voice	Begins to show some awareness of others' distress
B	Understands simple pronouns (e.g. *me, my, mine, he, him, his, she, her, hers*)	Uses simple negatives (e.g. *no, don't, not, none, nobody*)	Uses speech to achieve an outcome	Uses the vocabulary *happy, sad, angry* to describe pictures of faces
C	Understands the vocabulary and concept of *same* and *different*	Begins to use the conjunctions *and, but*	Uses language to make observations, share ideas and ask simple questions	Begins to show some empathy with others' distress
C	Understands common spatial prepositions (e.g. *in, under, on top*)	Use of pronouns is generally accurate	Uses simple language to express their own views and opinions	Says what makes me feel happy, sad or angry
D	Begins to respond to others in play contexts	Speech includes some adjectives to describe	With support, extends play to include some imagination	Shows awareness of a range of needs of others
D	Responds to simple instructions and directions from others	With support, initiates conversations and takes turns appropriately	Attempts simple explanations and answers simple problem-solving questions	Says what makes me feel excited or surprised

Suggested activities or strategies

Turn-taking

Taking turns forms the basis of all communication. Children who are stressed and who may fear others' language use because it may not be understood often want to take control and find it hard to allow another person to have their turn. It is often easier to explicitly teach and practise turn-taking through other activities.

Always do the activities in stages:
- you play just with the child;
- the child invites another to join in, so three of you take turns;
- you watch while the two children play;
- more children are invited to play; you watch;
- children play without supervision.

Each of these stages should be in place for several sessions, and the child should be happily allowing the other person to have their turn before you move on to the next stage.

- Play age and developmental-stage-appropriate board games which involve turn-taking.
- Use puppets and small world characters to enact age-appropriate social scenarios.
- Introduce a 'speaking object' – only the person holding the object is allowed to speak.

What is missing?

- Talk about objects and activities that are concrete for the child: *'What would you do if your water bottle was empty?'*; *'What can you do if you want to play with someone?'*; *'Are you ready to read?'* *'If not, what's missing?'*
- Use photographs of children and ask questions like: *'What if it was summer? How would her clothes change?'*; *'What's missing in this kitchen?'*
- Use packs of picture cards that have been created for *What if?*, *What's missing?* or *What's wrong?* questions, or search online for images.
- Do 'odd one out' and 'find three differences' puzzles in comics and puzzle books. Throughout, ask the child to say answers, not just point and circle.

Role-play

Role-play is a powerful way of improving a child's use of language for different purposes. Use the same stages (you and the child, add a friend, you supervise children, children play) as shown in the 'Turn-taking' section above. You may wish to use puppets or small world characters to make the activity more objective.

Create scenarios based on events that have recently happened in class. Always model the types of language you want the child to use. If the child was involved in a difficult situation themselves, you play the part of them in your role-play and ask them to play the part of an adult or another child.

After the role-play, identify and label the different purposes of language used. Was there arguing, explaining, discussing, negotiating, expressing emotions, etc.? Begin to make a list of the kinds of language used for the different purposes.

Emotional literacy

Emotional literacy is the ability of a child to 'read' and self-regulate their emotions and to recognise those emotions in others. Many studies show that it is critical for children's mental health.

- Reading and discussing stories together. Use developmental-stage-appropriate picture books if you can so children can begin to link expressions and body language with feelings. Talk about how a character felt, why they felt that way and how they show their feelings.
- Watch cartoons together. Talk about how a character felt, why they felt that way and how they show their feelings.
- Reflect their feelings back to the child. Comment on the emotions shown by the child by saying *'I think you're feeling happy now. You have a huge smile on your face. What makes you feel so happy?'* In this way, you help the child to link the word with the way they feel.

Aspect 3: Auditory processing for communication

Aspect 3: Auditory processing for communication

Letter	Receptive language	Expressive language	Semantics and pragmatics	Social communication
E	Thinks about what others are saying and comments on their ideas	Spoken language is intelligible, even out of context	Has an understanding of cause and effect, action and consequences	Looks at pictures and predicts whether someone is speaking in a quiet or loud voice
E	Understands comparisons	Regular past tense forms are generally accurate	Speaks of imaginary/fantasy situations using language such as 'Pretend...'	Looks at pictures and explains why someone might be speaking in a quiet or loud voice
F	Processes instructions containing four information carrying words	Begins to use complex sentences joined by 'because'	Begins to separate fantasy and reality	Uses vocabulary *worried* and *frightened* to describe pictures of faces
F	Tracks meaning and responds appropriately to eight-word sentences	Speaks in 5-6 word sentences	Laughs at visual slapstick humour	Says what makes me feel worried or frightened
G	Responds appropriately to a wide range of questions	Understands conversational conventions (e.g. turn-taking, maintaining a topic, interrupting)	Language use extends beyond communication to provide a basis for learning	Uses non-verbal signals of kindness, support and friendship
G	Asks for clarification if they don't understand	Uses a range of conjunctions, adverbs and prepositions to link ideas (e.g. *so*, *then*)	Accepts that people have different opinions in discussion	Looks at photographs and identifies body language associated with anger and aggression
H	Follows more complicated and abstract reasoning	Makes and expresses logical relationships	Uses problem solving and reasoning to complete a task or solve a problem	With support, uses words instead of actions to show anger
H	Understands a range of sentence types in context, including passives	Solves problems, explaining reasoning	Speaks of possibility (e.g. '*I hope*', '*I wish*', '*When I grow up*')	Displays characteristics of 'active listening' during a conversation

Suggested activities or strategies

Word webs

Children's vocabulary underpins their learning. The majority of children learn vocabulary almost incidentally as they hear words spoken around them and begin to explore the use of those words. Children with hearing difficulties, APD and often poor working memory may not have picked up these words as young children and may well have vocabulary and conceptual gaps. They will need to be taught vocabulary explicitly.

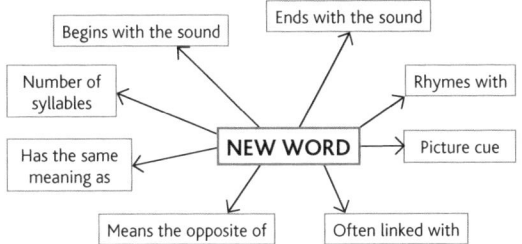

Word webs are an ideal way to develop vocabulary and to model ways of storing and retrieving new vocabulary.

The boxes in a word web can change according to the type of word but you should always include phonological information (the sound structure of the word) as well as semantic information (word meaning) as well as a picture cue. Storing all of this information will help children to retrieve the word more easily.

Extending sentences

Play games with sentences. Ideally, these should be written using words children can read because the child doesn't then have to remember the whole sentence while they're thinking about the conjunction (joining word). If children are not yet reading, write the sentence, drawing little pictures above verbs and nouns.

Once you have your base sentence, (e.g. *The king had to have toast for breakfast*) start adding conjunctions (e.g. *and, but, so, because, when, if*) and asking the child to complete the sentence. Talk about the fact that the way the sentence continues will depend on the conjunction (e.g. *because the cook forgot to buy cereal; and it made him cross; but he had some jam*, etc.).

Scaling feelings

On a piece of card, create a scale from 1–5. You can either use it to scale all feelings, or focus on one feeling the child struggles to manage (e.g. anger, anxiety, frustration). If you are scaling anger/anxiety/frustration, colour numbers 1–2 green, 3 yellow and 4–5 red, otherwise, let the child choose a colour for each number.

- As you reflect back to the child how you think they're feeling, use the scale to show a visual (e.g. 'I think you're feeling 5 for happiness because you've just done an amazing forward roll.'; 'I think you're feeling 4 on your anxiety scale because you're looking very worried about the spelling test.').
- Increasingly, ask the child to rate themselves on the scale and tell you how they know that's what they're feeling (e.g. they have a headache, their hands want to make fists, their tummy feels all bubbly). Learning to match physical feelings with an emotional state is the first step towards self-regulating.
- Once a child is able to scale their own feelings teach them some simple strategies which may enable them to manage the feeling (e.g. deep abdominal breathing, taking their weight on their arms, scribbling, having a sensory break in an agreed quiet place).

Hopes and wishes

Encourage the use of speculative language, even if you do it in silly ways (e.g. 'I wish I could swim in a bowl of jelly.').

- Have discussions inspired by books/films.
- Talk about what they'd like to do/be in the future. It doesn't matter how realistic their ideas are, it's important that children have aspirations.
- Make a list of character traits or superhero powers you both admire. Ask the child which one they would most like to develop. Ask them to think about:
    - what would change if you were ...?
    - how would you know you were ...?
    - what would you be able do that you can't do now?
    - how would other people know that you were ...?

Aspect 3: Auditory processing for communication

Letter	Receptive language	Expressive language	Semantics and pragmatics	Social communication
I	Uses contextual information to understand and learn new words	Describes objects and people using a wide range of adjectives	Shows interest in games with rules	Begins to link actions and emotions
I	Appropriately responds to all types of questions relating to familiar events or ideas	Begins, continues and ends a conversation appropriately	Begins to understand humour and may gather and repeat jokes and silly rhymes	Uses appropriate eye contact during conversations
J	Responds to complex questions relating to remote events	Uses grammatically correct sentences of 6–8 words	Knows that words can have more than one meaning (e.g. *row* can be a verb or a noun) and these are used in jokes	Responds to others' emotions and behaviours
J	Enjoys the social aspect of games and activities	Tries out new words to refine meaning and improve vocabulary	Enjoys puns and riddles and other language play	Recognises others' expressions, linked to their emotions
K	Talks about words and sentences to improve understanding	Corrects own vocabulary and syntactical errors	Begins to respond to sarcasm used in a jocular way	'Reads' body language to extend understanding of words
K	Recognises and understands metaphors and similes	Tries out figurative language such as similes and metaphors	Changes communication style for peers, family and adults in school	Recognises non-verbal signals of teasing and inappropriate social behaviours
L	Plays games that may have evolving rules	Argues logically, building on the previous speaker's ideas	Matches the seriousness/humour of a social situation	Understands what bullying is and knows that all forms of bullying are unacceptable
L	Knows some idioms and understands the concept	Uses language for multiple purposes including giving information, entertaining, persuasion and arguing	Adjusts speaking rate, voice, pitch, volume and intonation to match the context	Uses appropriate body language to match the context

Suggested activities or strategies

Idiomatic language

Many children struggle to grasp idiomatic language (e.g. *It was a piece of cake*; *It's a small world*; *The ball's in your court*; *Cross your fingers for me*; *I'm only pulling your leg*; *Hang on*) Children who take language literally inevitably find idioms particularly hard to grasp. There are lots of commercial products which help to familiarise children with idioms, but sometimes it's easier to make your own.

- Start with a list of up to 6–10 idioms that the child has heard.
- Cut A4 card into eighths and write an idiom in coloured pen on one piece of card and its meaning on another together with the child's drawing to represent the meaning.
- Use the pieces of card to play games such as:
  - **matching:** how quickly can the child match all of the idioms to their meanings?
  - **memory game/Pelmanism:** put the pieces of card in a grid formation. Take it in turns to turn over two cards. If you have the idiom and its meaning, keep the pair. If not, remember what you saw and the next person turns over two pieces of card.
  - **Lotto:** distribute the meanings cards between the players. One person then turns over the idioms cards and the player who has the meaning cards – and who can match the idiom to its meaning – places the idiom card face down on top of its meaning.

Using language for many purposes

Find or download short non-fiction texts with a range of purposes.

- Read the texts with the child: can the child identify what the purpose of each text is? How do they know? What are the clues?
- When might you need to use each of the conversational purposes to persuade, to entertain, to inform, to argue, to negotiate, to instruct and to bargain? Create a list of possible scenarios in which each distinct purpose would be useful (e.g. to persuade the teacher to extend Golden Time; to bargain with Mum that if I do this piece of homework, I won't have to do something else; to teach someone how to play a game).
- Let the child choose a scenario, but you get to choose which of the characters in the scenario you want to be. Tell the child that they need to try their hardest to achieve the conversational purpose, whether they are being the child or the adult in the conversation.

Speech prosodies and body language

When you have to concentrate on what the words and sentences are, it's all too easy to forget about pitch, tone, speed, volume and intonation but these prosodies carry a lot of information. It's a particularly challenging difficulty if the integration between left and right hemispheres isn't well developed because prosodies are processed in the right hemisphere, whereas the words are processed in the left hemisphere. The right hemisphere is also dominant for showing and understanding emotions through body language and facial expression.

- Activate the relevant part of the right hemisphere through listening to music with the child and talking about the mood of the music: angry, busy, sleepy, tender, etc. Help the child to identify the pitch, volume, speed and tone of the music. Can they stand and move in response to the emotion of the music?
- Watch cartoons with the sound turned down. Ask the child to predict from the action so far and the characters' body language what the speed, volume, pitch, intonation and impact of the voice is likely to be.
- Look at pictures in comics, picture books and online. Ask the child to predict from the character's expression and stance what the speed, volume, pitch, intonation and impact of the voice will be. Can they guess what the character might be saying?
- Agree some surreptitious signals that you will give to show the child that they are using speech prosodies, facial expression and body language appropriately or inappropriately.

Aspect 4: Auditory memory

Letter	Recall	Listening and remembering	Instruction processing	Sequencing
A	Remembers 2–3 words (or numbers) heard	Listens to a story from a picture book for up to 5 minutes with 1–2 other children	Follows a familiar instruction with up to two parts (e.g. 'Put your book in the pile and sit down.')	Recites short familiar rhymes
A	Recalls the first word in a three-word phrase	Participates in short conversations (2–3 exchanges)	Follows simple instructions to sort, categorise or match objects	Talks about own immediate experiences
B	Orally identifies the common sound heard in a tongue-twister	Responds to questions to identify objects (e.g. 'Which one do we sit on?')	Follows a familiar instruction with up to three parts (e.g. 'Put your coat on your peg, put your book bag in your drawer then sit down.')	Talks about past experiences
B	Counts backwards from three	Participates in short conversations (4–5 exchanges)	Processes unfamiliar instructions containing 1–2 information carrying words	With support, sequences three photographs of a recent activity
C	Repeats three words, or digits, in the order heard	With support, demonstrates understanding of basic conversational conventions (turn-taking, maintaining topic, not interrupting)	Follows a 1–2 step instruction when items/objects are present	Understands concept of past, present and future events in school day (e.g. 'We have done the register, now we're listening and next you can play.')
C	Concept of 'one more than' developing	Participates in conversations with one other person lasting 1–2 minutes	With support, participates in familiar games with simple rules	Able to imitate longer sequences such as classroom routines through play
D	Repeats two words or digits in reverse order	Listens to a story from a picture book for up to 10 minutes in a small group	Follows a 1–2 step instruction when items/objects are not present	Has some understanding of cause and effect, action and consequences
D	Orally blends three sounds to make a word	Listens to a story from a picture book for up to 10 minutes in a larger group	Processes instructions containing 2–3 information carrying words	Uses pictures to retell two events from a short, familiar story in sequence

Suggested activities or strategies

Information carrying words

Information carrying words (ICWs), also known as 'key words', are the words in an instruction that a child needs to understand in order to respond appropriately.

- If you and a child are sitting at a table, and on the table is a ball, a teddy and a cup, and you point to the ball, hold out your hand and say '*Give me the ball*', there are no information carrying words because you have given the child all the visual cues they need to pass you the ball.
- However, if you hold out your hand, without pointing to the ball and say '*Give me the ball*', the child needs to understand *ball* (1 ICW).
- If you don't hold out your hand, or point to the ball and say '*Give me the ball*', the child needs to understand *Give* as well as *ball* (2 ICWs).
- If you are sitting with a third person and you don't hold out your hand or point to the ball, when you say '*Give me the ball*', the child needs to understand *me* (as opposed to the third person) as well as *give* and *ball* (3 ICWs).
- When you count the information carrying words in an instruction, you need to consider the context in order to decide how many of the words the child must understand in order to carry out the instruction.

Once the principle is established you can use activities with only a few ICWs across the curriculum. Activities you can try include (nouns, verb, adjectives and prepositions are included as examples only):

- 1 ICW: have the objects/pictures in front of you and ask questions like '*Give me the ball*' or '*Where is the ball?*'
  ○ have a large box on the floor and ask the child to '*Get in the box*', '*Go around the box*'.
- 2 ICWs: have the objects/pictures in front of you and give instructions like '*Point to the ball*' or '*Put your finger on the ball*';
  ○ '*Give me the red ball*' (where there is a choice of red or blue balls and you hold out your hand);
- 3 ICWs: '*Put the ball in the box*' (where there is a choice of a box and a basket and the ball could go on or in the box);
  ○ '*Colour the big box blue*' (where the child has some colouring pencils and some pictures of different-sized boxes to colour).

Sequencing

- Sequencing pictures:
  ○ ask the child to sequence 2–3 photographs of themselves doing/making something;
  ○ then ask the child to sequence 2–3 pictures/photographs of other children doing/making something;
  ○ next, show two pictures and ask the child to predict the third;
- give the child experience of taking simple oral messages to other children, other adults in the room, other adults in the school;
- give the child 2–3 instructions with sequencing words introducing instructions with 1–2 ICWs, e.g.:
  ○ '*First get your writing book*;
  ○ *then get a pencil*;
  ○ *then sit on your chair*.'

Remember, think, say

- Auditory working memory for learning involves three processes:
  ○ recalling the information;
  ○ processing the information;
  ○ communicating the information.

We can give children opportunities to practice developing these processes by asking them to listen to a list of words and to repeat the list in reverse order so that words are processed, not simply recalled. The words can be digits (e.g. *three*, *seven*, *four*), letters (e.g. *p*, *f*, *e*) or nouns/verbs (e.g. *mouse*, *rain*, *brick*). Digits are easier because there are only ten possible options; there are a total of 26 possible letters and possibilities of nouns or verbs are endless.

It is important, even at the early stages, to ask children to use the strategies in genuine situations such as orally blending or segmenting a word, remembering which items have been counted or remembering the beginning of a sentence when you're reading words at the end of it.

Aspect 4: Auditory memory

Letter	Recall	Listening and remembering	Instruction processing	Sequencing
E	Counts up to ten scattered objects, remembering what has previously been counted	Begins to use strategies to work out a partially heard word	Follows three-step instructions when items/objects are not present	Sequences and repeats three pieces of heard information in a message or instruction
E	Orally segments a CVC* word	Remembers simple inferential meanings (e.g. 'Who's talking?' means 'be quiet.')	Processes instructions containing 3–4 information carrying words	Uses pictures to retell three events from a short, familiar story in sequence
F	Remembers common maths facts (e.g. 2+2=4; 5+5=10)	Understands common abstract ideas such as *same/different* and *more/less*	Remembers and delivers a simple message	Retells three events in sequence from a story or personal experience from memory
F	Repeats 3–4 words or digits	Listens to teacher talk with visual support for 10 minutes	Uses a visual task chart to follow new 3–4-step instructions	Plans activities using a sequence of three ideas or actions
G	Blends sounds heard to identify a picture or object of a CCVC (e.g. *f-r-o-g*) or CVCC (e.g. *t-e-n-t*) word	Answers concrete *wh-* questions about a short passage from a book or shared experience	Processes instructions containing four information carrying words	Time concepts are developing to include a *tomorrow, next week, next year* as well as *yesterday, last week, last year*
G	Recalls sentences of 5–7 words	Participates in simple discussion about a book or shared experience	Uses a visual task chart to follow new 5–6-step instructions	Predicts what might happen next in a story
H	Blends sounds heard to identify a picture or object of a CCVCC or CCCVC word (e.g. *g-r-ou-n-d* or *s-t-r-i-ng*)	Understands and responds to all common question types in context	Follows four-step instructions	Names times of the day associated with an activity (e.g. '*We listen to a story at home time*')
H	Counts on to and back from numbers to ten to solve mental arithmetic questions	Asks the teacher/other speaker for clarification about immediate events if needed	Shows interest in games with rules (such as sports)	Tells short stories containing at least three elements of 'story grammar' (e.g. *setting, characters, time, plot*)

*C = consonant   V = vowel

Suggested activities or strategies

Modelling maths

A good working memory is essential to mental maths: you have to remember the original problem even as you retrieve the maths facts you need to do the calculation and manipulate the information to find the answer.

- Model solving a similar problem before you ask the child to do it. This will remind them of the processes.
- If more than one process is needed, colour-code them as you model them so the child has a visual memory cue.
- Make sure children have access to table-top information that will help them to retrieve necessary maths facts.
- Give children opportunities to overlearn maths facts and processes. Children with weak auditory memories need more practice in order to store the information in long-term memory and retrieve it quickly and easily.

Draw it out

Many children find visual information easier to recall than spoken. If you explicitly teach children how to jot down images while you are talking or giving them problems to solve, they will learn how to apply the strategy successfully.

- Maths problems, including mental maths problems, are easier for children to understand when they are represented visually.
- Children may find a 100 square easier to visualise than a number line. Just jotting down the numbers they need, showing the relationships as shown on a 100 square, may provide enough information for children to understand how to proceed.
- Give children alphabet arcs so they can develop familiarity with where in the alphabet a letter lies.
- Demonstrate drawing family trees so children can understand relationships between rulers, monarchs, or their own extended family.
- Teach them to make sketch maps so they can begin to understand relationships.
- Introduce a range of graphic organisers (mind maps, KWL grids, SWOT analysis – find any

others that are useful) and let children write/draw on them as you talk.

Too much to do

Before a child begins an activity, make a visual task chart with them showing how the activity can be broken down into smaller chunks. The task chart should be drawn quickly to show the separate stages of the activity (e.g.:

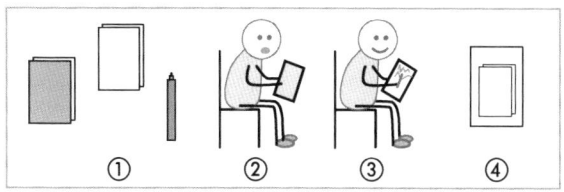

① Get your reading book, your English book and a pencil.
② Read the next part of your reading book.
③ Answer the questions in your writing book.
④ Put your writing book in the 'finished work' tray.)

Increasingly, expect the child to help you to decide what to represent on your task chart.

Wh- words and stories

Introduce, or remind the child, of the wh- question words: *who, where, when, what, why, how*.

- Explain that all stories need to have information that relate to each of the words – probably more than once.
  - Characters = *who*
  - Setting = *where/when*
  - Problem = *what/why*
  - Exciting bit = *what/how*
  - Solution = *why/how*
- Put the words on the table and begin to tell a familiar story to the child. Ask the child to pick up the *wh-* words which are relevant to what you have said.
- Swap roles so that the child retells the same story and you pick up the *wh-* words.
- Once the child is confident, begin to make up stories, based on those the child has read, and ask the child to pick up the *wh-* words.
- Swap roles.

Aspect 4: Auditory memory

Letter	Recall	Listening and remembering	Following instructions	Sequencing
I	Orally blends or segments words with 4–5 sounds into component phonemes (e.g. *s-t-r-ea-m*)	Makes logical relationships from information heard	Learns and applies new rules for a familiar game	Answer questions about the plot in a story
I	Identifies differences between pairs of heard CVC* words (e.g. *pat, pack*; *pat, cat*; *pat, pet*)	Links new information to what is already known	Asks questions to clarify expectations	Answers questions about the order of events in a story
J	Identifies differences between CVC words and similar CVCC/CCVC words (e.g. *bed, bend*; *fog, frog*)	Asks questions to clarify what is being said	Listens carefully to instructions and remembers the points	Predicts events that might occur after a story has finished
J	Remembers most number bonds of and to ten	Listens to a short chapter of a book read aloud (no pictures) and answers questions	Repeats instructions accurately	Explains the sequence of main actions in a chapter from a book
K	Explains how you change a word to make a new one (e.g. *tap* into *tape* or *trap*)	Listens to teacher talk for 20 minutes	Begins to negotiate rules of a made-up game (e.g. tag)	Gives clear instructions for playing a game
K	Recalls and repeats 3–4 words or digits in reverse order	Compares new information to what is already known	Follows instructions given to the class which refer to immediate actions	Uses visual prompts to include information about *who*, *what*, *when*, *where*, *why* and *how* in recounts and narratives
L	Blends and segments to read and spell at age-appropriate level	Processes information and learns when only verbal information is given	Follows instructions given to the class to improve abstract ideas such as outcomes or behaviours	Uses a wide range of conjunctions, adverbs and prepositions appropriately
L	Recalls taught number facts and uses them to solve simple problems	Asks and answers appropriate questions during whole-class teaching sessions	Follows instructions given to the class which refer to more distant or abstract actions, behaviours or objects	Recounts experiences in appropriate sequence and detail

*C = consonant   V = vowel

Suggested activities or strategies

Listening comprehension activities

There is a wide range of books which include listening comprehension activities where children are asked to look at a picture and add objects/colour objects/draw objects. Some even promote curriculum skills like maths, phonological awareness or spelling. These can be useful because they:

- break up listening with doing;
- give support for extended periods of concentration;
- can be done with a group or a class so that no child feels different;
- help children to pay attention to the important words in an instruction;
- help children to prioritise actions based on understanding;
- gradually increase the complexity of the demands on the child.

As with all other interventions, these activities will only increase children's ability to listen, attend and follow instructions if you build on the skills throughout your school day and across the curriculum, including referral to past and future events and actions.

Barrier games and activities

Barrier games are activities where two children sit opposite one another with some kind of barrier between them (which could be a file, a hardback book or a small whiteboard) so that neither can see what the other is doing. Children have identical resources. The idea is that one creates/constructs/draws something while giving instructions to the listener to enable them to create the same outcome. The listener may have to ask questions to clarify details.

- Begin with simple coloured 2 x 3 grids and a range of small objects. The speaker needs to use language such as '*Put the blue counter on the red square*'.
- Move on to non-coloured grids and objects which may need adjectives to describe them (e.g. '*Put the large green brick on the top left hand square*'). (You may need to indicate left and right on the grid.)
- Other activities include threading beads, constructing simple models, creating pegboard or geo-board patterns.
- Drawing activities such as adding details to maps of drawing simple shapes are much harder and involve more explicit language in both questions and answers.

Number facts

Number facts should be overlearned in isolation before being used to solve problems. Overlearning should be secure at each stage of the following progression:

- initially give simple number bond questions in a familiar format (e.g. 4 + 6 = …);
- then keep the question simple, but change the way the question is asked (e.g. '*What do I add to 4 to make 10?*');
- continue to keep the questions simple as you use more demanding vocabulary (e.g. '*What is the difference between 4 and 10?*');
- once the child is accurate, and the answer is retrieved fairly easily, begin to use the number facts in problem solving (e.g. '*Jenny needs £10 to buy a game. She has saved £4. How much more does she need to save?*').

Until the number facts are easily recalled, ensure that the child has access to table-top resources (such as tables squares or lists of number bonds or tactile resources).

Show and tell

Once children are able to retell familiar stories and to adapt stories they know to create their own variation, challenge them to use what they have learned when recounting personal anecdotes. They will need to:

- think about the *wh-* words they need to include in their recount: *who, when, where, what, why, how*;
- identify background information their audience needs in order to create the context;
- prune unnecessary information, so they only focus on what is important in the retelling;
- consider how much detail the audience needs to know and when to include it;
- think about where to begin and end their anecdote.

Aspect 5: Visual-spatial memory

Letter	Matching and remembering objects	Matching and remembering shapes and symbols	Matching and remembering location	Matching and remembering patterns
A	Remembers one item from a photograph or picture	Matches a shape to a picture of the shape	Points to the *first* car/person/animal in a queue of three	Places shapes to match a row of three given
A	Remembers two items from a photograph or picture	Matches a picture to a related symbol	Points to the *last* car/person/animal in a queue of three	Places shapes to match a row of four given
B	Remembers how many of a given item were in a picture (up to two items)	Finds a shape of the same colour as the one shown from a choice of three	Points to the *top* object in a tower of three objects	Orders two pictures on the basis of *now* and *next*
B	Remembers how many of a given item were in a picture (up to three items)	Finds a shape of the same size as the one shown from a choice of three	Points to the *bottom* object in a tower of three objects	Orders three pictures on the basis of *first*, *next*, *last*
C	Remembers two attributes of an item shown (e.g. colour and shape)	Makes three pairs of picture cards from a choice of six picture cards	Look, cover, say, check: says which object in a tower of three was *at the top*	Look, cover, place, check: places two objects in the order shown
C	Remembers three attributes of an item shown (e.g. colour, size and shape)	Makes three pairs of shapes from a choice of six shapes	Look, cover, say, check: says which object in a tower of three was *at the bottom*	Look, cover, place, check: places three objects in the order shown
D	Answers simple questions about an object viewed for 30 seconds	Makes three pairs of shapes or symbols from a choice of six shapes or symbols	Look, cover, say, check: says which car/person/animal in a queue of three was *first*	When shown the first two pictures from a familiar sequence of three, can predict the final one
D	Answers simple questions about an object viewed for 20 seconds	Finds a shape of the same colour and size as the one shown from a choice of three	Look, cover, say, check: says which car/person/animal in a queue of three was *last*	When shown the first and last picture from a familiar sequence of three, can predict the middle one

Suggested activities or strategies

Digital photographs
Use a simple digital camera to take pictures of classroom objects, as well as children doing routine sequences of actions (e.g. hands are dirty, wash them, dry them; tidy away, return to your seat, sit quietly; put on artwork apron, do artwork, remove apron). Use your pictures for many of the visual memory activities (but be aware of your school's Acceptable Use policy and avoid using personal mobile phones).

Naming
Children with weak visual memories often have stronger verbal ones. Whether or not this is the case, the children will benefit from having additional 'memory threads' as they talk about and name what they see.

- When you show the child an object or picture, allow them to talk about it while they look at it and perhaps handle it. Ask prompt questions while the child is looking at the object to seek information about colour, size, shape, texture, use *reminds you of …*'
- Ask the child to take a mental photograph of the object. Can they 'see' the object/picture if they shut their eyes?
- Only after talking about it and naming it should you hide the object/picture and ask questions about it.
- As you ask your questions, ask child to shut their eyes and 'see' the object/picture.

Matching, sorting and categorising
Matching, sorting and categorising are key skills which underpin a lot of learning.

- Matching is finding two or more identical objects, recognising an object from, for example, its picture or the sound it makes.
- Sorting is using one or more attributes of different objects (e.g. colour, shape, size, material).
- Categorising is identifying something according to a more abstract grouping (e.g. how it's used, type of creature, type of clothing, etc.).

These are critical skills for the ways in which we store and retrieve words, ideas and memories. Children with additional learning difficulties, such as autism, often struggle with categorising because one object can belong to more than one category (e.g. an apple could be categorised with things that begin with *a*, red things, things that grow, food, fruit, 'things I like to eat', etc.).

Matching is more important than sorting or remembering in the early stages of remembering shapes and symbols (including letters and numbers).

- Initially, use tactile shapes/symbols rather than pictures of them so the child can explore with touch as well as vision.
- Give the child a shape/symbol and ensure that the objects you place on the table for the child to match their shape/symbol to are very different (e.g. if you want the child to find another letter *g*, show them *m*, *t* and *g*).
- Talk about the shape/symbol and emphasise the quality that is important for the activity.

Look, cover, do, check
As children begin to engage with memory activities, introduce the sequence of *look, cover, do, check* to embed the expectation that they self-assess and correct if necessary. This sets up useful skills for:

- copying words or text;
- reading comprehension;
- retelling stories;
- looking again at answers in maths activities.

Sequencing cards
- Teach children to sequence two and then three picture cards. Model telling the stories/explaining the sequence and ask the child to repeat it.
- Use sequencing words *first*, *then/next*, *last/finally* and encourage the child to do the same.
- Show them any two cards of a familiar sequence in order. Can they remember what the missing card shows?
- Show them any two cards of a new sequence in order. Can they predict what the missing card shows?

Aspect 5: Visual-spatial memory

Aspect 5: Visual-spatial memory

Letter	Matching and remembering objects	Matching and remembering shapes and symbols	Matching and remembering location	Matching and remembering patterns
E	When playing Kim's Game, remembers two related objects	Makes a collection of shapes with a shared attribute	Look, cover, place, check: orders two items in the order as shown	Describes a two-step repeating pattern
E	When playing Kim's Game, remembers two unrelated objects	Makes a collection of shapes which match a picture viewed for 10 seconds	Look, cover, say, check: identifies which item is missing in a queue of three	Continues a two-step repeating pattern
F	When playing Kim's Game, remembers two objects from the same category	Sorts shapes into groups according to one attribute	Points to the *first*, *second* and *third* item in a queue of three	Look, cover, place, check: copies a two-step repeating pattern
F	When playing Kim's Game, remembers three objects from the same category	Makes a collection of shapes according to two attributes	Adds a *first*, *second* or *third* item to an initial queue of two objects	Creates a new two-step repeating pattern based on one seen previously
G	When playing Kim's Game, remembers two objects from the same category and an unrelated object	Matches symbols from a choice of three	Look, cover, place, check: adds the third item to join two already in correct sequence	Describes a three-step repeating pattern
G	When playing Kim's Game, remembers the object that is not related to a category	Matches symbols from a choice of four	Look, cover, say, check: places three items in correct sequence viewed for 10 seconds	Continues a three-step repeating pattern
H	When playing Kim's Game, identifies something that has been added	Look, cover, point, check: identifies the same symbol from a choice of two	Look, cover, place, check: places three items in the location as shown on 2 x 2 arrays	Look, cover, place, check: replicates a three-step repeating pattern
H	When playing Kim's Game, identifies something that has been taken away	Look, cover, point, check: identifies the same two symbols from a choice of four	Look, cover, say, check: names the location as shown on 2 x 2 arrays viewed for 10 seconds	Creates a new three-step repeating pattern based on one viewed previously

Suggested activities or strategies

Kim's Game

Kim's Game can be played in a number of ways, but always involves the child looking at a range of objects, the objects being covered and the child remembering some aspect of what they saw. As well as increasing the number of objects, the complexity can be altered by:

- using objects that are related to each other (e.g. knife, fork) rather than unrelated objects (e.g. fork, gluestick);
- moving the position of one or more object;
- adding an object;
- removing an object;
- equalising spaces between objects having added/removed an object;
- naming all the objects when placed in a grid;
- naming all the objects when placed in a line;
- naming the first/second/third, etc. object in a line;
- naming all the objects when placed randomly in a space.

Making linear patterns

We need to recognise and remember patterns of letters to read, patterns of numbers to understand place value and multiplication tables and patterns of events to predict what might happen next. Copying, describing and extending patterns, as well as creating new patterns, is an important step in learning. Look for patterns in the environment as well as making patterns using:

- counters, cubes or beads for threading;
- pegboards and geoboards;
- pens, crayons and collage materials;
- construction toys;
- 2D and 3D shapes;
- numbers, letters and abstract symbols.

Lines and queues

Use toys, cars and small world animals and people to make lines and queues to reinforce ordinal vocabulary and memory.

- Ask the child to name (or describe an attribute of) each object in the queue.
- Cover or hide the queue.
- Ask the child to *either* name all of the objects from memory *or* name the first/second/third or last object in the queue.

Letters, numbers or symbols

Make a line of 2–4 letters, numbers or symbols from left to right. Check the child knows where the line begins (at the left hand side) and ends (at the right hand side).

- Ask the child to name (or describe an attribute of) each letter, number or symbol.
- Cover or hide the line.
- Ask the child to match one or two of the letters, numbers or symbols by looking at a set of 2–4.

Using arrays

As well as asking children to remember location in linear sequences, ask them to remember items placed in grids or arrays.

Begin by using 2 × 2 arrays, then increase to 2 × 3/3 × 2 and 3 × 3. You and the child should have replica arrays for each activity. Initially, place one object on the array and ask the child to copy and place their item in the same cell. Then ask them to:

- place objects to recreate the top row/bottom row;
- place objects to recreate the first column/second column;
- place all the objects as shown on the original grid.

Once the child is confident at placing items, begin to use look, cover, place, check: the child looks at the array you have completed, you cover your array while the child places the objects in replica cells. The child then checks for accuracy.

Increase the challenge by:

- considering the relationship between the objects; very different objects may be easier to recall than similar-looking objects;
- using symbols and shapes where the child has to consider more than one attribute as well as the location of the object.

Aspect 5: Visual-spatial memory

Aspect 5: Visual-spatial memory

Letter	Matching and remembering objects	Matching and remembering shapes and symbols	Matching and remembering location	Matching and remembering patterns
I	When playing Kim's Game, identifies two items that have been added	Matches a symbol that is facing left or right	Look, cover, place, check: adds a fourth object to join three already in the correct sequence	Describes a four-step repeating pattern
I	When playing Kim's Game, identifies two items that have been taken away	Matches a symbol that is pointing up or down	Look, cover, place, check: orders four objects in the order as shown	Continues a four-step repeating pattern
J	When playing Kim's Game, identifies two items that have been swapped over in a line	Look, cover, say, check: remembers whether a symbol was facing right or left	Look, cover, say, check: names the position of requested four items in a 2 × 2 array	Look, cover, place, check: copies a four-step repeating pattern
J	When playing Kim's Game, identifies two items that have been swapped over in a random array	Look, cover, say, check: remembers whether a symbol was pointing up or down	Look, cover, say, check: lists all four items in a 2 × 2 array	Creates a new four-step repeating pattern based on one viewed previously
K	Plays Pelmanism (pairs) using 12 cards (6 pairs) in a 3 × 4 array	Look, cover, point, check: remembers and matches one attribute of a symbol or shape including orientation	Look, cover, point, check: identifies the item that was in a specified place in a 3 × 3 array	Look, cover, place, check: recreates a pattern of three symbols pointing up or down
K	Plays Pelmanism (pairs) using 12 cards (6 pairs) in a random array	Look, cover, point, check: remembers and matches two attributes of a symbol or shape, including orientation	Look, cover, point, check: identifies the item that was in a specified place in a 3 × 3 array	Look, cover, place, check: recreates a pattern of three symbols facing left or right
L	Plays Pelmanism (pairs) using up to 20 cards (10 pairs) in a 5 × 4 array	Look, cover, point, check: remembers and matches one attribute in a row of four similar symbols or shapes	Look, cover, point, check: identifies two items that were in specified places in a 3 × 3 array	Look, cover, place, check: recreates a pattern of four symbols pointing up or down
L	Plays Pelmanism (pairs) using up to 20 cards (10 pairs) in a random array	Look, cover, point, check: remembers and matches two attributes in a row of four similar symbols or shapes	Look, cover, point, check: recreates a 3 × 3 array	Look, cover, place, check: recreates a pattern of four symbols facing left or right

Suggested activities or strategies

Remembering sequences

The ability to remember visual sequences will help children to use and make their own visual timetables and task managers. Using and making these visual supports gives children more independence in the classroom.

- Show images of a familiar four-step sequence, using photographs, pictures, words or commercial sequences which cover activities like:
  - getting up;
  - getting ready to leave the house;
  - arriving at school in in the morning;
  - preparing to learn;
  - getting changed for PE/swimming;
  - getting changed after PE/swimming;
  - organising belongings at dinnertime;
  - what we do when the bell rings at the end of playtime;
  - getting ready to go home.

Select sequences which are important to the child – either in school or at home –and with which they need help.

- Talk through the sequence and check the child's understanding of each step before changing focus to memory activities.

Memory game/Pelmanism/pairs

There are many commercial versions of the game, and a range of online and digital games, some of which are free. They are all the same insofar as:

- pictures are placed face down on a surface;
- players take it in turns to reveal two pictures. If they are a pair, the player keeps them, if not all the players look at the cards which are then turned face down again and play continues;
- the winner is the player with most pairs at the end of the game;
- the challenge is always to remember the images revealed by other payers in order to make pairs yourself.

The game can be made easier or harder by:

- the number of pairs of cards: 8 cards (4 pairs) is probably the smallest number needed to play a game;
- the similarity of the images: finding pairs of faces is harder than finding pairs of unrelated images;
- the relationship between the images: it's harder when the pictures are different angles/fractions of the same objects: it's hard matching pictures of quarters of an apple when distractor images show whole apples, half apples and apple cores;
- how the cards are laid out on the playing surface: grids (e.g. 12 cards set out in rows of 4) are easier than lines which are easier than cards laid randomly).

Remembering direction

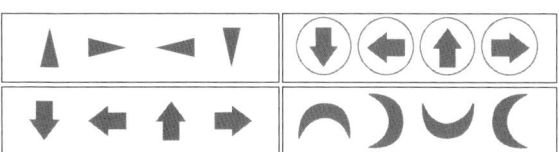

Use pictures of arrows, road signs, isosceles triangles placed on their bases, sides and point, as well as other shapes, to increase the difficulty in matching and remembering in lines or grids. Make computer images and take digital photographs showing:

- shapes – and shapes inside shapes – in different rotations;
- plane shapes in different rotations;
- place settings with knives and forks pointing up, one up one down, and both down;
- any other resources which are familiar but which you can use to show direction.

Use your images to make all games and activities more complex and demanding.

Aspect 6: Kinaesthetic memory

Letter	Copying movements	Copying symbols	Hand-eye co-ordination	Handwriting
A	Visually tracks a ball or toy as it moves across a floor	Makes horizontal marks on a page with some control	Makes more than one horizontal mark on a page	Places pencil on page near a marked point
A	Visually tracks a ball or toy as it moves towards and away along a floor	Makes vertical marks on a page with some control	Makes more than one vertical mark on a page	Places pencil on page on a marked point
B	Visually follows a finger or pen as it moves across a page	Draws broadly circular shapes, moving clockwise with some control	Colours a large shape with horizontal, vertical and circular marks	Moves pencil from one marked point to another across, up or down a page
B	Visually follows a finger or pen as it moves around a page	Draws broadly circular shapes, moving anti-clockwise with some control	Colours largely within borders of a large shape with horizontal, vertical and circular marks	Moves pencil from one marked point and returns to roughly the same place
C	Visually follows a finger or pen as adult draws long horizontal lines	Makes marks that cross the body's midline randomly	Makes repeated marks that cross the body's midline randomly	Draws 5 cm lines vertically and horizontally between 1.5 cm spaced parallel lines
C	Visually follows a finger or pen as an adult draws long vertical lines	Makes marks that cross the body's midline vertically	Makes repeated marks that cross the body's midline vertically	Draws a 5 cm curved line between 1.5 cm spaced curved lines
D	Visually follows a finger or pen as an adult draws long diagonal lines from top to bottom	Makes marks that cross the body's midline diagonally, from top to bottom	Makes repeated marks that cross the body's midline diagonally, from top to bottom	Traces vertical lines of different lengths
D	Visually follows a finger or pen as an adult draws long diagonal lines from bottom to top	Makes marks that cross the body's midline diagonally, from bottom to top	Makes repeated marks that cross the body's midline diagonally, from bottom to top	Traces horizontal lines from left to right

Suggested activities or strategies

Tracking

A child's ability to move around the school and around a classroom relies on them successfully tracking where their peers are and where there are obstacles in their way. The ability to track objects with eyes only, or with head-rotation and eyes is particularly fundamental to the development of literacy and numeracy skills: we track progression of letters through a word, of words across and down a page as we read and write, and we track when using number lines, number squares and multi-digit numbers in maths. You can improve eye-tracking skills by:

- starting by using balloons and slow moving objects before moving gradually to smaller and smaller balls rolled across and along wide spaces
- running your finger under words as you read aloud to the child, expecting the child's eyes to follow your finger
- showing photographs and pictures and exploring the child's understanding of perspective: are they aware that the people in the distance are not just smaller than those in the foreground?
- drawing a box on a computer screen. Change your cursor into a mouse/aeroplane/racing car or other interesting shape and ask the child to follow it with their eyes as you move it around the screen. Can the child say '*stop*' when you move the cursor into the box? Gradually decrease the size of the box.

Crossing the midline

This refers to the ability to reach across the middle of the body. You need it, for example, to draw a line across a piece of paper without having to swap hands in the middle or to sit cross-legged on the floor. Try:

- placing a drum on either side of the child; challenge the child to reach across their midline to play the drum with the hand on the other side of the body
- using masking tape to make a bendy track with sharp corners on the floor. Give the child a toy car and ask them to push the car along the track. Increase the challenge by asking them to do it with one hand behind their back, or make the track into a rough octagonal shape around the child and ask them to push the car using one hand, then the other.
- placing containers to one side of the child and small objects to sort into the containers on the other side
- lie on the floor beside the child. You both need torches. Play torch-tag across the ceiling, with one torch light following and trying to catch the other.
- using streamers to make big, long, shapes in the air
- sitting or standing opposite the child and teaching them to play pat-a-cake games, clapping their hands against yours. Increase the challenge by including pat-a-cakes where their left-hand claps against your right hand.
- placing a large sheet of paper in front of the child. Draw lines the length of the paper with a coloured marker pen.
- giving the child a stamper in each hand and ask them to make a line of stamps using alternate hands.

Get creative

- Give the child experience of using a range of colouring materials, including paint, crayons, felt pens, gel pens and coloured pencils as well as painting and colouring programmes on the computer. Work co-operatively to colour pictures. Model different ways of moving your hand to colour larger and smaller areas. Talk about the advantages of thicker and thinner pens and brushes. Also discuss colour choices.
- Make thick strips of corrugated card and ask the child to paint them.
- Make different shapes using playdough: roll the dough to make snakes and balls and use rolling pins and cutters. Try dough disco moves to encourage the child to use all their fingers to make small indents and deep holes and to prod, poke, stretch, squeeze, bash the playdough (there are a lot of video clips and instructions for dough disco online).

Aspect 6: Kinaesthetic memory

Aspect 6: Kinaesthetic memory

Letter	Copying and tracking movements	Copying and tracking symbols	Copying and tracking lines	Handwriting
E	Traces long and short horizontal and vertical lines	Uses eye-tracking to predict where an adult will end a horizontal or vertical line	Traces and continues a pattern of long and short vertical or horizontal lines	Copies vertical lines and horizontal lines from left to right
E	Look, cover, draw, check: long and short vertical and horizontal lines	Traces horizontal lines with a right-angled change of direction, having watched an adult draw them	Traces and continues a pattern of long and short vertical and horizontal lines	Traces horizontal and vertical lines with right-angled change of direction
F	Traces squares and rectangles	Copies and draws two intersecting lines to make a horizontal cross shape	Traces and continues a turret pattern with three turrets	Traces letters: *i* and *l*
F	Copies while an adult draws: squares and rectangles	Copies while an adult draws a horizontal cross shape	Copies while an adult draws a turret pattern with three turrets	Look, cover, write, check: letters *i* and *l*
G	Traces diagonal lines from top left to bottom right and from bottom left to top right	Copies and draws two intersecting lines to make a diagonal cross shape	Traces and continues a pattern of *v* shapes	Traces letters: *v, w, x, z*
G	Look, cover, draw, check: diagonal lines from left to right	Joins simple dot-to-dot shapes and patterns with diagonal lines	Traces and continues a zigzag line with four points	Look, cover, write, check: letters *v, w, x, z*
H	Traces curved lines and circles	Joins simple dot-to-dot shapes and patterns with curved lines	Traces and continues a pattern of curves	Traces letters: *t, u, j, y*
H	Copies while an adult draws curved lines	Copies while an adult draws curves facing different directions	Colours inside the edge of round shapes mostly within the line	Look, cover, write, check: letters *t, u, j, y*

Suggested activities or strategies

Posture

Handwriting is a whole body activity, not simply restricted to the fingers. A good posture for handwriting includes:

- two feet on the floor to balance the body
- hips slightly higher than knees so the weight is more on the feet than the back;
- bottom at the back of the chair so the lower back is supported;
- straight back, but leaning slightly forwards;
- non-writing arm resting on the table so that the body's weight is balanced.

Consider:

- the height of the chair. If the child's feet don't touch the floor, can you provide a solid step for them to rest their feet on? Or do you need to borrow furniture from a class of younger children?
- the height of the table should be at the child's elbow height so the elbow rests comfortably on the table.

Pencil grip

Look at the child's pencil grip. If they are not using a well-balanced tripod grip, consider why not.

- The most common reason for children to complain of pain when writing is that too much pressure is exerted on the pencil by the forefinger of the writing hand. Watch while the child writes: is the forefinger bent down at the top knuckle? If so, remind them to make the top knuckle flat or slightly raised. This gives more comfort and more flexible fingers.
- Don't let left-handed children develop a hooked wrist, curving above the line of writing. Encourage left-handed children to tilt their paper to the right so that the edge of the paper is parallel to their forearm.
- If you have concerns about a child's pencil grip, consider:
  - using a silicone or rubber pencil grip (see www.ldalearning.com for a wide range of different grips);
  - offering a triangular or ergonomic pencil;
  - referral to an occupational therapist.

Tracing and templates

Make use of activities like:

- tracing pictures;
- drawing round temple shapes;
- using cut-out areas to guide the pencil;
- looking online for pencil control activities to print off or manage onscreen;
- looking in comics and puzzle books for simple mazes.

Staging dot-to-dots

Dot-to-dot puzzles are excellent for children who have visual-motor integration problems (including hand-eye co-ordination) because dot-to-dots require visual tracking ahead of the pencil as well as following the marks making.

- Choose or make simple dot-to-dots which need lines of the sort you are practising. If necessary, share different parts of the puzzle, so you do some, leaving the child with the focus line shape.
- You need two copies of the picture.
- Use a yellow highlighting pen to draw the lines you want the child to trace.
- Let the child trace your line.
- Give them another copy of the dot-to-dot without your highlight line for them to complete independently.

Looking at circles and curves

Where do we see circles and rings in the environment? Go on a curve and circle hunt around the school making lists of circles and curves (e.g. clocks, footprints, cups, water bottles, containers, flowers, playground markings, 0s, letter *c, s, o*, etc.).

- Place tracing paper/greaseproof paper over simple line drawings of circles and curves.
- Use finger paint to paint over patterns of circles and curves.
- Practice circular wrist movements by threading nuts and bolts, turning keys in locks, stirring flour and water.

Aspect 6: Kinaesthetic memory

Aspect 6: Kinaesthetic memory

Letter	Copying and tracking movements	Copying and tracking symbols	Copying and tracking sequences of symbols	Handwriting
I	Look, cover, draw, check: a square or rectangle with four sharp corners	Joins simple dot-to-dot shapes and patterns with diagonal lines	Look, cover, draw, check: a sequence of three squares (large, small, large)	Traces letters: r, n, m, h, b, p, u
I	Look, cover, draw, check: a triangle with three sharp corners	Joins simple dot-to-dot pictures with a range of lines	Look, cover, draw, check: a sequence of three triangles (large, small, large)	Look, cover, write, check: letters t, u, j, y
J	Copies while an adult draws a circle	Joins simple dot-to-dot shapes and patterns with diagonal lines	Traces a sequence of three squares (large, small, large)	Traces letters: c, a, d, g, o, q, s, f
J	Look, cover, draw, check: a circle	Joins simple dot-to-dot pictures with a range of lines	Traces and continues a pattern of different-sized circles (large, small, large)	Look, cover, write, check: letters c, a, d, g, o, q, s, f
K	Look, cover, write, check: capital letters with straight lines A, E, F, H, I, K, L, M, N, T, V, W, X, Y, Z	Look, say, cover, write, check: a CVC* word ...	... and at increasing speed, on dots spaced in regular spaces along a line	Writes known words with most letters sitting on a baseline (ascenders and descenders shown)
K	Look, cover, write, check: capital letters with curves B, C, D, G, J, O, P, Q, R, S, U	Look, say, cover, write, check: a word with four letters	Places their pencil accurately, and at increasing speed, on dots placed randomly on a page	Writes a CVC word, leaving appropriate spacing between letters
L	Look, cover, write, check: numerals	Look, say, cover, write, check: a number with four digits	Traces within the lines of simple straight line mazes	Writes known words with regular and controlled lower and upper case letters
L	Writes any letter or numeral from memory	Look, say, cover, write, check: a word or number with five or more letters	Traces within the lines of simple curved line mazes	Writes more than one word, leaving appropriate spaces between words

*C = consonant   V = vowel

Suggested activities or strategies

Letter formation and handwriting

Teach letter formation carefully and gradually, emphasising the letter families and shared movements between them.

Check the child:

- starts all letters (except *d* and *e*) at the top;
- does the 'bounce back' along the original pencil line.

Once letter formation has been taught:

- insist it is used in *all* writing, not just in handwriting or intervention sessions;
- correct bad letter formation before it becomes habitual;
- don't compromise and accept rushed work because you're grateful the child has done something. In the longer term, the child is likely to develop an aversion to all writing if their handwriting is illegible.
- as children look, say, cover, write, check words, use a checklist to reinforce what good handwriting looks like.

Securing letter shapes

Make letter shapes fun by reinforcing with activities such as:

- give the child a vibrating pen to copy or trace letter shapes – the additional sensory input will help to secure the letter formation skywriting, Make a large letter shape – or sequence of letter shapes – in the air. Can they:
  - say which letter(s) you made?
  - copy the letter(s) by skywriting?
- if the child is happy to be touched and gives their permission, write the letter(s) on their back or the palm of their hand. Can they say and skywrite the letter(s)?
- write letters in a range of tactile substances, e.g. sand, sugar, icing sugar, flour, salt, rice, shaving foam, cornflour and water mix. (Colleagues in Reception classes are likely to have everything you need for this activity.)

Capitals and numbers

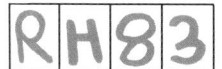

Give the child opportunities to practise writing capitals and numbers in upright rectangular shapes. This will help to reinforce the size to height ratio as well as help to maintain consistency in size and height.

Writing words

Don't attempt to write any words unless the child is confident at segmenting and blending: it is expecting too much to combine a focus on the sounds in the word as well as the letter formation and reading. If sounds are not secure, focus instead on numerals or patterns of shapes.

Think about the child's progress in phonics: only ask them to write words they can read in order to emphasise that the purpose of writing is communicative.

The look, say, cover, write, check procedure should be used consistently.

- Begin with two-letter words (e.g. *as, at, if, in, it, on, no, be, do, go, me, to, we*).
- Move on to three-letter CVC words (e.g. *bus, den, jog, kit, let, mop, net, van, wax, zip*).
- Move on to four-letter words with short vowels (including words such as: *best, cook, just, lost, mint, nest, plan, quit*).
- Finally, progress to four-letter words with long vowels (e.g. *boil, claw, dice, fast, gone, hail, join, lane, moon, nose, part, vote, wine, hoax, zoom*).

Mazes

- Look in children's comics and puzzle books for mazes.
- Find puzzles which involve tracking wavy, intersecting lines to join objects, letters or numbers. Ask children to track the lines with eyes, fingers or by tracing them in different colours.
- Draw a curved maze on thin card. Place a small magnetic shape above the card and a magnet below it. Can the child lead the shape around the maze using the magnet underneath the card?

Aspect 7: Memory, attention and organisation

Letter	Attention	Planning	Organisation	Prioritising
A	Gaze and attention is responsive to movement and noise in the environment	Matches pictures to resources	With adult support, puts own belongings away	Selects a preferred activity from a choice of two
A	Wears ear defenders in noisy environments	Uses individual pictures to collect resources	With picture support, puts own belongings away	Identifies a preferred book from a choice of two
B	Manages normal classroom noise without ear defenders	Responds to picture cues to follow routines and rules	With support, follows familiar classroom routines	Responds to picture cues to follow routines and rules
B	Puts hands over ears to request ear defenders	Collects two resources when shown two pictures	Puts coat on before gloves or hat	Holds simple classroom responsibility
C	Focuses for 3 minutes on a self-chosen activity	Responds to three picture photo sequences to collect resources	Puts finished work in an identified place	Selects a preferred activity or book from a choice of three
C	Responds to own name being called when focused on a self-chosen activity	Knows language *now* and *next*	Follows a sequence of three pictures to tidy objects away	Follows an adult direction to focus on named items in a picture
D	Focuses for 5 minutes on a self-chosen activity	Knows language *first*, *second* and *third*	Knows that a timer shows how much time is left	Responds to *now* and *next* cards
D	With support, shifts their focus to an adult speaker, then returns to a self-chosen activity	Knows that activities can be broken down into stages	With support, takes their clothes off for PE in an appropriate order	Knows that good or bad choices have consequences

Suggested activities or strategies

Comfort and safety

Before we can expect children to pay attention, plan, organise and prioritise we need to ensure that are comfortable and that they feel safe. We can help them by:

- ensuring that they have their toileting needs met;
- checking that they are neither hungry nor thirsty;
- ensuring that they are sitting with good balance on stable seats so their feet touch the floor;
- ensuring that they can see us easily without craning their necks;
- giving them the freedom to shift their weight to avoid numbness and soreness;
- developing good relationships so the children feel that we care about them and they don't fear us;
- making sure lighting is appropriate – no glare of light into their eyes;
- checking that they can hear adequately with minimal background noise;
- making sure that the classroom is appropriately heated/ventilated;
- giving each child enough personal space without crowding;
- keeping our teacher talk time to a minimum. (Children can concentrate for their age in minutes +/– 2, so an eight-year-old can be expected to concentrate for between 6 and 10 minutes.)

Picture that

As the child gets undressed for PE:
- name each item of clothing;
- use sequencing language of *first*, *then*, *next*, *after that*, *finally*, etc. as you prompt them or ask questions such as 'What will you take off next?';
- if the child gets stuck, help them to take off most of the items (e.g. take the sock down over the heel) but let them finish taking each garment off. 'Backwards chaining' like this allows the child to feel as if they were successful. Next time, you can let them do more of the job themselves.
- encourage the child to make a neat pile of the clothes so they know which order to put them back on again;
- take photographs of the pile of clothes as each garment is added to it. Before the next lesson, print out the photographs and work with the child to sequence them in order to create a visual timeline of the process.

Create a choice board

Create a choice board on a piece of card and laminate it so you can use it several times.
- The box at the top is for the context.
- The boxes in the middle row show good and bad choices.
- The boxes in the bottom row show the consequences of the good and bad choices.

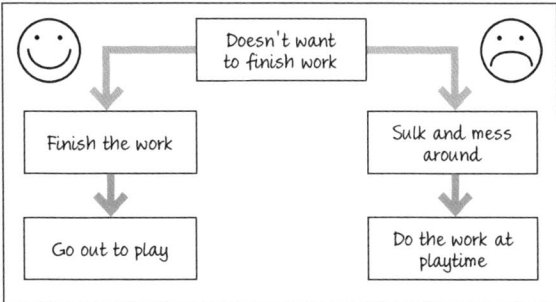

It is important that children learn to choose and to prioritise their behaviour in the secure knowledge that every behaviour has a consequence but some are good and some are bad.

Make sure that the consequences are consistent with the school's behaviour policy and don't penalise a child if they have a disability or learning difficulty.

Aspect 7: Memory, attention and organisation

Letter	Attention	Planning	Organisation	Prioritising
E	With warning, manages own response to loud noises	With support, responds to an instruction to wait for 15 seconds	With support, puts clothes on, taking from the top of a pile	Selects a preferred activity from the choice available
E	Focuses for 10 minutes on a self-chosen activity	Collects two resources given only oral instructions	Response to instructions to move *fast* and *slow* in PE	Selects a preferred book from the choice available
F	Controls the focus of attention between an adult- and a self-chosen activity	With support, responds to an instruction to wait for 30 seconds	With support, begins to do activities in an allocated time	Responds to *now*, *next*, *later* cards
F	Independently refocuses attention on a self-chosen activity	With support, looks at a 'job chart' to identify own jobs in the classroom	With support, begins to do activities more slowly and carefully	Independently identifies the important elements in a picture
G	Focuses for 10 minutes on an adult-chosen activity	Works with others to collect resources for a group project	When reminded, looks at a timer for a cue to speed up or get ready to move activities	With support, identifies stressful situations and discusses options
G	When own name is called, listens to what an adult is saying, without stopping a familiar activity	Puts clothes into a neat pile to show the order they need to be put back on	Follows taught organisational routes such as *Get ready*, *Do*, *Done*	Accepts consequences for bad choices
H	Focuses on an adult voice even when the classroom is noisy	With support, responds to an instruction to wait for 1 minute	Starts a task within 3 minutes of being asked	Says what they like and dislike about choices given
H	Focuses for 15 minutes on an adult-chosen activity	Puts hand up before speaking	Looks at a timer for an indication of time left and responds appropriately	With support, identifies simple goals

Suggested activities or strategies

Curriculum organisers

Many children find boxes reassuring – they contain and limit the expectations in terms of quantity of work to be completed. Children with sensory integration difficulties may need to be taught explicitly how to approach a task methodologically – working from left to right and top to bottom. Consistent layout and organisation of curriculum support structures enables children to have a reliable base for managing their workload.

- Use writing frames with a brief description of what should be recorded in each box (e.g. *introduce the character and the setting; begin the action; make this part exciting; what happened next?; how did the story finish?*).
- Use maths problem frames (e.g. *underline the important words; which operation will you use: +, −, ×, ÷?; estimate what you think the answer might be; write the calculation; write the answer*).

Ensure that the child has the chance to talk through the activity and clarify each stage before they begin. Thereafter, expect them to work as independently as possible.

Think it, say it

Create simple Think it, Say it cards to show that some ideas should only be thought and others can be spoken. Use the cards as prompt cards to remind children when it is appropriate to speak during whole-class time or guided group work.

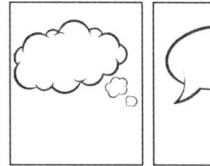

Think it, Say it cards can be used to help children to identify what it is appropriate to say out loud and what it better just to think.

Think, pair, share

Use the same cards in think, pair, share to ensure that all children feel that their voice is heard by someone.

Think: everyone thinks about what they have just learned or thinks quietly about the answer to a question.

Pair: everyone turns to their response partner and tells them what they were thinking. In this way, everyone's thoughts are voiced and heard, even if not by the teacher.

Share: people put their hand up and wait. If their name is called, they can share their ideas with the whole class (but not everyone can share their ideas with the whole class).

Using timers

Timers are a very strong asset and can be used flexibly according to the learning behaviours of the children in your class to:

- build in rest breaks after a certain point in the activity (e.g. *'When you have done 10 number sentences, turn the time over and you can read your book until it runs out.'*);
- increase the challenge (e.g. *'Yesterday, you were able to do an activity in x number of minutes. Can you beat that time today?'*);
- facilitate transitions (e.g. *'In three minutes we're going to stop our maths and tidy up. Then it will be music.'*);
- speed up a slow child (e.g. *'The timer is about half way. You should have finished cutting out your pictures and sticking them in order. Now you need to write a sentence about each one.'*)

Self-assessment

Self-assessment is an important life skill so we know what we need to do better in order to improve. Support the child to self-assess their work and identify some goals.

- Choose one or two statements from a task's success criteria. (If relevant, select criteria which are linked to previous targets.)
- Consider each of the statements separately. Can the child tell you what 'success' would look like and where they have achieved it?

Aspect 7: Memory, attention and organisation

Letter	Attention	Planning	Organisation	Prioritising
I	Listens as part of a group for 10 minutes	Works in a group to plan a shared project	With support to prioritise actions, increases the pace when requested	Identifies stressful situations and discusses options
I	Listens to what an adult is saying while concentrating on an activity	Uses a list (words or pictures) and collects resources	With support, self-assesses outcomes against expectations	Identifies goals for activities and actions
J	Manages own response to unexpected loud noises	Breaks an activity into manageable chunks	Looks at an analogue clock for an indication of time	Identifies potentially stressful situations and plans for options
J	Listen as part of a class or group for 15 minutes	Identifies items that will be needed for a future activity	Tells the time at o'clock, half past and quarter past	With support, picks out information in a more selective manner
K	Shuts out distractions and remains focused	Independently, collects book bag and all belongings at the end of the day	Knows when a task is finished and the goal has been achieved	Filters out unwanted information
K	Listen as part of a class or group for 20 minutes	Organises self to prepare to come to school	Independently moves on to the next stage of an activity	Uses sticky notes and highlighter pens to colour-code prioritisation
L	Pays focused attention in a group or class for the duration of a lesson	Completes activities and meets expectations	Accurately estimates the time needed to complete an activity	Concentrates on essential aspects of information
L	Takes responsibility for reactions to unexpected loud noise	Uses lists, planners and timetables to plan and check	Starts and finishes tasks within an allotted time frame	Securely identifies priority actions and information

Suggested activities or strategies

Support for planning

Teach the child a range of different ways of planning so they can identify and begin to use the ones that work for them. Try:

- **planners**: these are generally used to record homework and things to remember to bring to school tomorrow. If the homework is more than a few words long, print it off for the child to stick in their book or ask someone else to write it in. At the very least, ask someone to check that it's been copied correctly.
- **calendars**: use calendars that show a month on one sheet of paper so the child can plot the pattern of activities over a period of time and see how long it is until an anticipated event;
- **timetables**: if the child can read them, give them a copy of your timetable and highlight each subject in a different colour;
- **sticky notes**: some children like to make lists on sticky notes and discard their notes when the matter has been dealt with.

Managing reactions

Some people may react more fearfully than others to certain situations, but make it clear that we are all responsible for managing our own reactions.

- Use a choice board (see page 79) to identify consequences of different reactions.
- Ensure that the child knows the full range of acceptable options available to them – which may need to include leaving the room for a while until anxiety is reduced.
- If the child finds ear defenders are helpful, ensure they are easily and quickly available. If they are not available, discuss alternative ways of reducing the impact of sudden loud noises (e.g. by covering the ears tightly with the hands).

Managing time

Many children – particularly disorganised children – find the concept of time hard to grasp and yet school days are ruled by the need to be on time. You can help the child by:

- supporting them in keeping their working environment and tray/locker as well-organised and decluttered as possible. Build in weekly opportunities to tidy and declutter.
- offering support during the 'about to begin' phase of the activity in order that the child can be as independent as possible for the duration of the task;
- ensuring that resources are easily available – provide some additional sharpened pencils so the child doesn't have to waste time sharpening their pencil;
- having clear routines and expectations so the child knows what to expect;
- providing visual or verbal tick lists or task charts (see page 63) for the child to tick off each stage of the activity;
- giving regular warnings throughout the activity so the child knows that they are progressing at an appropriate pace;
- preparing children for changes in routines.

Prioritising

Prioritising requires us to understand:

- the overall goal;
- the time available;
- prioritising the main sections within the task;
- monitoring progress towards the goal.

As children try to prioritise the main sections help them to think in terms of:

- I **can only** achieve my goal if I (e.g. have a book; have someone to help me to access to the internet; write three sentences);
- it **would be good** to (e.g. draw pictures to show what I have found out as well as writing use colour to write my sentences).

Agree that the **can only** statements are those that take priority.

Help the child to construct a plan for an activity, for example:

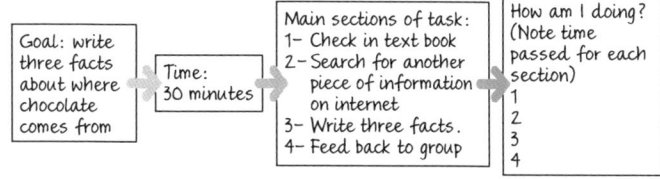

Aspect 7: Memory, attention and organisation

References

Alloway TP (2007). Automated working memory assessment (AWMA). Oxford. Pearson. www.pearsonclinical.co.uk

Alloway TP, Gathercole S & Kirkwood H (2008). Working memory rating scale. (WMRS). Oxford. Pearson. www.pearsonclinical.co.uk

Baddeley A (2000). The episodic buffer: a new component of working memory? *Trends in Cognitive Sciences*. 4 (11): 417-423.

Baddeley A, Eysenck MW & Anderson MC (2015). Memory. 2nd edn. Hove & New York. Psychology Press.

Blank M, Rose SA & Berlin LJ (1978). The language of learning: the preschool years. New York. Grune & Stratton.

British Society of Audiology (2011). Position statement: auditory processing disorder (APD). Reading. British Society of Audiology. www.thebsa.org.uk/wp-content/uploads/2014/04/BSA_APD_PositionPaper_31March11_FINAL.pdf

Children and Families Act 2014. London. HMSO.

Department for Education & Department for Health (2014). Mental health and behaviour in schools: departmental advice for school staff. London. HMSO.

Department for Education (2015). Special educational needs and disability code of practice: 0 to 25 years. London. HMSO.

Gathercole SE & Alloway TP (2007). Understanding working memory: a classroom guide. London. Harcourt Assessment.

Gathercole SE & and Alloway TP (2008). Working memory and learning: a practical guide for teachers. London. SAGE Publications.

Great Ormond Street Hospital (2014). Auditory processing disorder (ref: 2014F1485). London. GOSH NHS Foundation Trust.

Sirimanna T & Grant P (2016). Auditory processing disorder. www.cafamily.org.uk/medical-information/conditions/a/auditory-processing-disorder

Turner M & Risdale J (2004). The digit memory test. Dyslexia International. www.dyslexia-international.org/content/Informal%20tests/Digitspan.pdf

Links to other *Target Ladders* titles

Target Ladders: Dyslexia
Kate Ruttle

Includes additional targets for:
- Phonological awareness;
- Phonics and spelling;
- Reading comprehension and fluency;
- Planning, organising and remembering.

Target Ladders: Visual Perception
Mark Hill

Includes additional targets for:
- Visual memory;
- Visual sequential memory.

Target Ladders: Speech, Language and Communication Needs
Susan Lyon et al.

Includes additional targets for:
- Attention control;
- Comprehension;
- Expressive language;
- Social communication;
- Phonological awareness, auditory discrimination and speech.

Other useful resources from LDA

Short Term Memory Difficulties in Children
Joanne Rudland

Working Memory and learning – A Practical Guide for Teachers
Susan E Gathercole and Tracey Packlam Alloway

How to Understand and Support Children with Visual Needs
Olga Miller and Karl Wall

I hear with My little Ear (Books 1 and 2)
Liz Baldwin

For more resources suitable for children with visual perception differences, visit www.ldalearning.com